Praise for

THE TELOMERE MIRACLE

"I have known Dr. Park since 2010. I met him while working on my book *Bombshell*. Reading *The Telomere Miracle* deepened my understanding of physiology and inspired me. Dr. Park has an open mind and a big heart and that's what makes his book not only easy, but really fun to read."

— **Suzanne Somers**, actress, singer, entrepreneur, and *New York Times* best-selling author

"This vividly written book is very interesting not only by its the popular scientific consideration of how we can personally influence our health for the better, but also by its analysis of many facts concerning aging. Highly recommended reading."

— **Alexey Olovnikov, Ph.D.**, scientist and Nobel Prize nominee

"Dr. Park's insights and collaboration have been invaluable to our company. His ability to explain complex systems in a clear way is a unique gift. Telomere erosion is a central driver of illness and aging. This book explains how the process works and also delves deeply into the aspects of lifestyle that can mitigate this damage."

— **Stephen J. Matlin**, CEO of Life Length

THE
TELOMERE
MIRACLE

ALSO BY ED PARK, M.D.

Telomere Timebombs
Maximum Lifespan

THE TELOMERE MIRACLE

Scientific Secrets to Fight Disease, Feel Great,
and Turn Back the Clock on Aging

ED PARK, M.D.

HAY HOUSE, INC.
Carlsbad, California • New York City
London • Sydney • Johannesburg
Vancouver • New Delhi

Published and distributed in the United States by: Hay House, Inc.: www.hayhouse .com® • *Published and distributed in Australia by:* Hay House Australia Pty. Ltd.: www .hayhouse.com.au • *Published and distributed in the United Kingdom by:* Hay House UK, Ltd.: www.hayhouse.co.uk • *Distributed in Canada by:* Raincoast Books: www .raincoast.com • *Published in India by:* Hay House Publishers India: www.hayhouse .co.in

Cover design: Christopher Tobias • *Interior design:* Pamela Homan
Interior illustrations: Cecelia Snaith
Indexer: Joan Shapiro

Library of Congress Cataloging-in-Publication Data

Names: Park, Edward, (Dr.) author.
Title: The telomere miracle : scientific secrets to fight disease, feel
   great, and turn back the clock on aging / Ed Park, M.D.
Description: Carlsbad, California : Hay House, Inc., [2018]
Identifiers: LCCN 2017034165 | ISBN 9781401952570 (hardback)
Subjects: LCSH: Telomerase. | Aging--Molecular aspects. |
   Telomerase--Pathophysiology. | BISAC: HEALTH & FITNESS / Alternative
   Therapies. | HEALTH & FITNESS / Healthy Living. | MEDICAL / Genetics.
Classification: LCC QP606.T44 P36 2018 | DDC 612.6/7--dc23 LC record available at
https://lccn.loc.gov/2017034165

Hardcover ISBN: 978-1-4019-5257-0
10 9 8 7 6 5 4 3 2 1

1st edition, January 2018

Printed in the United States of America

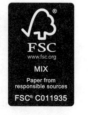

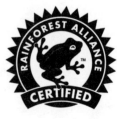

*To my patients: you are my greatest teachers
and the inspiration for all I do.*

CONTENTS

AUTHOR'S NOTE

If you're like me, you may not always read the introductory stuff before the actual book. I urge you to make an exception here; this book might prove to be a challenge without some contextual remarks.

I was once giving a talk at UCLA about my Telomere and Stem Cell Theory of Aging when a man interrupted to lob a question at me: "Since telomerase is active in cancer cells, won't taking telomerase activators *increase* cancer growth?" I began my reply, but the man simply stood up and walked out, so while the rest of the audience benefited from his question, he did not. I don't want this to happen to you.

I have found that my ideas sometimes make people angry. Most people resist questioning the status quo, groupthink, or dogma. Unfortunately, history has shown us that whether deductive, as in "How many angels can fit on the head of a pin?" or inductive, such as "As above, so below," our search for wisdom is hindered by mental laziness. It is just easier to accept whatever doctrine already exists than to question it. For example, if I cast doubt on the value of antioxidants, the superiority of certain diets or exercise regimens over others, or the inevitability of aging, you may feel upset because I am asking you to rearrange beliefs that are already set in your mind.

Why does this happen? Beliefs are how you make sense of the world, so they are not easily given up. Rare is the person who wants to hear what he doesn't want to hear. Let's imagine that you were adopted, but your parents never told you the truth. If I knocked on your door and told you of your adoption, you would probably think I was either crazy or a horrible person and would most likely dismiss the new information outright. The new idea is seen as a threat because it asks you to rearrange some pretty serious beliefs about how you understand your world. Granted, the example I've just used is extreme, but a similar response often occurs even when relatively mild shifts are proposed from our existing ideas and current understanding of how to stay healthy and disease free.

As a result of their own strong beliefs, people who read my website or blogs or hear my talks sometimes misconstrue my more controversial ideas as unjustified, frivolous, or exaggerated. I assure you, I don't consider anything in this book to be controversial, although my explanations are not yet widely accepted.

So why did I write this book, if I can already anticipate it may annoy you or make you uncomfortable?

1. To impart a deep and practical knowledge of the key systems that mediate aging, balance, and health in our bodies. This is your "quick-start" guide to how your body works.

2. To interpret the scientific literature regarding telomeres in many areas of health and wellness using my simple and unified Telomere and Stem Cell Theory of Aging.

3. To increase your mastery of what we'll call the "TeloMirror Tools" so that you can live a better life.

I am a medical doctor, blogger, video producer, and theorist who treats patients with strategies that enhance the body's own internal fountain of youth on a cellular level: TELOMERASE. This is the enzyme in our stem cells that reverses normal telomere shortening, which you will see is at the heart of all aging and disease. Within this book you will discover a new way to understand aging and disease that I believe will soon be regarded as common sense. After you read this book, you might be forlorn to realize that what seems obvious to you and me will still be considered speculative to the uninitiated for some time to come.

You will be introduced to scientific studies, presented with new paradigms of health and aging, so I hope that rather than being threatened by this, you may welcome the additional information as the powerful weapon against aging that it is. At the very least, even if you end up disagreeing with some of what you read, contemplating new and contrasting evidence to the opinions you hold dear can actually strengthen your position or refine it to a stronger and more nuanced one.

The simple yet profound message you'll find here is that inside your cells, your body already has the necessary tools to repair itself and to stay young forever.

There are hundreds of scientific studies linking telomere health with the six critical functions discussed in this book: breathing, mind-set, sleep, exercise, diet, and supplements. What's more, there are thousands of studies linking telomere dysfunction to nearly every disease known. I propose that the diseases can be precipitated or resisted depending on how well we optimize those six functions. My son Oliver coined the term *TeloMirrors,* which nicely captures this notion: telomere dysfunction in the research literature *reflects* the efficiency of natural repair of telomeres and cells. The literature strongly suggests that the healthier your telomeres, the less likely you are to have genetically damaged and dysfunctional cells and to manifest diseases, including the pseudo-disease of aging itself.

If you might forgive the mixing of metaphors, think of the six TeloMirror Tools (TMTs) as six cylinders in an engine, all doing their part to create force. There are no "bad" ways to push the crankshaft of wellness (see picture on page iv), just as there is no real "bad" way to breathe or sleep. But if each of the six areas both reflects and propels our wellness, we should strive to optimize each one of the TMTs to achieve maximal health, happiness, and healing.

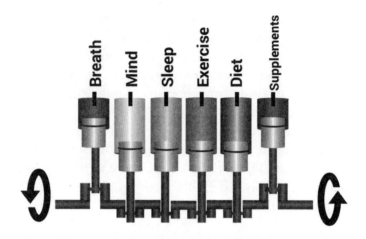

Perhaps you picked up this book because you have the nagging sense that there are simpler explanations about aging, wellness, and disease than those that are currently promoted. Many experts seem to be pushing anti-aging fads like game-show hosts, while the medical system seems fixated on the inevitability of decay. You don't have to agree with all of my ideas, but if you keep an open mind, I promise that you will learn new and useful ways to stay young. I invite you—unlike the man who walked out of my lecture—to stay put even when you become uncomfortable.

I won't offer up any universal cookbook of dos and don'ts. Instead, each of the chapters will invite you to master the basic principles of how these TMTs *function*, review the science linking telomere problems with *dysfunction*, and then use your wisdom to forge a plan to *optimize* how your own cylinders are firing. There is no guru, method, or teacher that will serve everyone; you will use your intuition to connect to your own truths by leveraging the knowledge within this book.

I suppose the purpose of this author's note is that I hope you won't stand up and walk out on me. My unified theory and some of my insights may occasionally stir up resistance in your mind, but I merely ask you to consider the possibility that illness and aging are constantly being created, resisted, and even cured in your body, and that growing old is something that may soon be vanquished completely with just a little help from science—and from your friends: breathing, sleeping, mind-set, exercise, diet, and supplements.

Could I be right?

Read on and decide for yourself.

NOTE: The information in this book must not be misconstrued as medical advice. Science, like your physiology, is complicated and dynamic and can never be reduced to a list of absolute dos and don'ts. Please consult with a physician before making changes in lifestyle to ensure they are compatible with your medical condition and any medications you require. If you experience any worrisome symptoms, consult your physician immediately.

PART I

AGING IS OPTIONAL

We'll begin at the beginning, of course. Chapters 1, 2, and 3 are designed to provide you with some background about my journey and then provide a crash course in cell biology and my unified theory of aging and disease.

The chapters in Part II will focus on the TeloMirrors of breathing, mind-set, sleep, exercise, diet, and supplements. After that, you'll achieve a profound understanding of each of the systems that you constantly use to maintain telomeres and resist aging and disease.

Finally, in Part III, we'll perform a self-assessment "tune-up" of your own engine of health. The book closes with a preview of what our bright future holds in store for us: living a healthier life well beyond what you currently might believe is possible.

Chapter 1

The Quest to End Aging

*Question all you believe and
believe only what you've questioned.*

Telomere, schmelomere—what's it all about?

If you follow the latest science news, you may already have heard about telomeres and how they are the key to a whole new way of understanding aging. Just in case you haven't, let's review: Telomeres (from the Greek: telo=end, mere=body) are protective caps of repetitive DNA (deoxyribonucleic acid) at the ends of all your cells' chromosomes.

Chromosomes are made up of specific sequences of billions of DNA molecules, assembled in matched parallel helical chains and then coiled up in the nucleus of the cell. DNA is the universal information coding system that somehow stores the directions for building and maintaining *you* and all life on earth, except some viruses. If the telomeres are

Telomeres

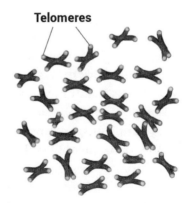

like blank tape leader in old cassettes, then the music is the DNA between the telomere ends.

The health and longevity of your telomeres is what holds the key to aging—or, more importantly, *not* aging. But the loss of telomeres is also associated with nearly every known disease. This is not merely a coincidence. You will come to understand that it is a direct, causal relationship.

Telomeres are needed for all plants and animals with linear chromosomes, though not needed for many bacteria, which possess circular chromosomes and hence have no ends to protect. Here's a quick picture to show you what this looks like:

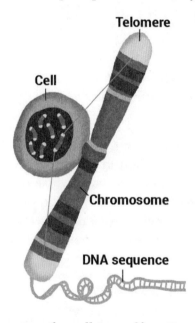

Telomere

Cell

Chromosome

DNA sequence

At this very moment, many of your cells are dividing. They do this to replace dead cells (you lose and replace tens of billions of cells every day). As we will explain in the next chapters, each time a cell divides, a little bit of the telomeres on the tips of your DNA cannot be copied, so eventually, the "blank tape leader" in the descendants of these dividing cells will shorten to the point of no longer protecting the music. Loss of the blank tape produces chromosome mutation, and this in turn causes the cell to malfunction and die. Why does it die? I'll get into this in depth in the next chapter, but for now, just know that your DNA is the musical score with the information for building and orchestrating the symphony of cells that make up your tissues, your organs, and their healthy cooperation.

To switch metaphors, I suppose you could say that telomeres keep chromosomes intact in the same way that fuses prevent firecrackers from exploding. When the fuse burns down and reaches the firecracker, it goes—BOOM. The same thing happens to your cells' chromosomes. When telomeres "burn" down, your valuable and precious DNA mutates and then the cell can't operate correctly because the operating instructions are damaged.

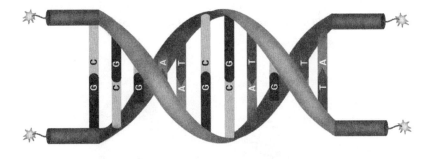

This is the primary mechanism of cell death and is a normal part of cell ecology for ordinary, non-stem cells.

Key point: telomere shortening is actively reversed only in special "master copy" cells known as stem cells, because they can relengthen their telomere fuses by using a special enzyme, or micromachine, called telomerase.

We'll unpack everything you need to know about stem cells in the next chapter. For now, just know that preserving the stem cells by keeping telomerase activity efficient holds the key to health and longevity as suggested by the scientific literature. Because all cells derive from stem cells, if you have old and damaged stem cells, you are going to have old and damaged regular cells.

For the record, while my simple interpretation is ignored by the majority of scientists, I believe that over time, aging is merely an emergent property caused by progressive shortening of telomeres in stem cells, which causes chromosome mutations. So, in a sense, you age because your stem cells age. Luckily, we are born with large reserves of stem cells and the capacity to protect them with telomerase, and all cells have mechanisms for self-destruction when they become damaged.

Simply put: If you were better able to preserve the telomeres in your stem cells, you'd better resist the aging process and reduce your risk of disease, because your DNA would remain protected for longer. Thanks to telomerase, you *can* do this. What may sound like science fiction to you is actually a scientific fact. **Telomerase is an enzyme working in your stem cells right now to regrow your telomeres.**

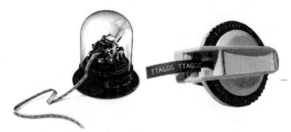

The Telomerase Enzyme adds back
more telomere length

What's more, telomerase is potentially active in every stem cell in every single plant and animal on earth, so this is certainly no obscure backwater of science. In recognition of this, three scientists were awarded the 2009 Nobel Prize in Medicine or Physiology for "the discovery of how chromosomes are protected by telomeres and the enzyme telomerase."[1]

Before you stand up and walk out on me, let me share the most incontrovertible evidence directly linking telomerase to aging that is real and scientifically well known: premature aging, or progeria.

Normally, healthy adults inherit two copies of nearly all genes (one from Mom's chromosome and one from Dad's). Genes are sequences of DNA "songs" that encode for specific proteins. Unlike all the other contrived theories of aging, we have many naturally occurring experiments from Mother Nature in which one parent gives a defective telomerase gene copy, resulting in what we call a "half gene dose" of telomerase. The result of having only one of two functional telomerase genes is known as clinical *progeria*— the accelerated aging condition resulting in teenagers dying from what is indistinguishable from regular "old age." With two copies of telomerase (a full gene dose), most of us can reasonably hope to survive into our 80s. But with more copies or more efficient usage of our normal two copies, who knows how long we could last? That is the point of this book.

The clues to my simpler and unified paradigm of aging are found everywhere in the vast and growing body of telomere research. Strangely, no one has dared to try to unify all these studies—until now. Enter my Telomere and Stem Cell Theory of Aging (fully explained in the next chapter). Once you comprehend this simple explanation, you will understand aging and illness as simply one disease with a thousand faces.

If you want to deeply understand the theory, you will need to spend some time understanding the basic biology of Chapters 2 and 3. But if you just want the "quick start" guide, you'll find that each of the chapters in Part II will explain physiology, present convincing evidence of a link between each TeloMirror Tool and telomerase activity, and suggest some best practices to optimize your telomerase activity using self-knowledge and mastery.

How did I come to believe all this? To explain how I arrived at my current understanding of aging as a condition incurable by current thinking, I need to take you back to an allegorical true story, back to 1991 and my very first night on call in a hospital as a green third-year medical student on his first clinical rotation. That peculiar night was the first of many lessons about birth, life, and death in my 26 years in clinical medicine. This almost fractal journey has taken me from student, to teacher, and then back to student many times: first as a practicing obstetrician and gynecologist and now as a consultant to those seeking mitigation for aging. I sometimes say, "I attended births earlier in my career, but now it's mostly rebirths."

TRIAL BY FIRE: FIRST NIGHT FORESHADOWS ALL

As medical students, we spend the first two years in classrooms and the last two years in hospital rotations. During my very first hospital rotation as a third-year medical student, I drew the short straw and got the first surgical night call (meaning I was on duty for the overnight shift). I was a bit nervous, but thought, *What's the worst that could happen?* I know now that this is never a wise question to ask the universe.

Only a few hours into my shift, I was called to the bedside of an elderly woman who was in obvious distress, and breathing rapidly, had a low blood pressure, and showed a tender and bloated abdomen. This particular woman had long suffered from Crohn's disease (a horrible autoimmune condition that basically rots your small intestine). She was recovering from her fourth bowel resection. It was obvious even to an inexperienced medical student like myself that she had probably suffered an intestinal rupture at the site of surgical repair and that her intestinal fluids were spilling into her abdominal cavity. I expected the team to rush her back to the operating room to repair her intestines.

Instead, the junior resident (my direct superior) checked with the senior resident (*his* superior), who then consulted the attending physician (aka the doctor of record). The junior resident told me that the plan was to "buff the chart," which is medical-speak for documenting the appropriate investigative actions without any heroic intervention. So, as directed, I drew the patient's blood, monitored her vital signs, ordered X-rays of her abdomen, and documented our findings. And—for the next two hours—I watched helplessly as this poor frightened woman writhed in agony. I stayed by her side; I held her hand; I tried to say reassuring words.

I hadn't ever seen someone die, so it wasn't until I checked and found no pulse, waved my hands in front of her open eyes, and got no response that I called out to the senior resident, "I think she's dead."

"What!?" he shouted.

There was a lot of scrambling, first to confirm my diagnosis and then to call a Code Blue (a cardiopulmonary resuscitation).

And then all hell broke loose.

In rushed the anesthesiologist to force-ventilate the patient with a handheld bag; I straddled the patient's chest and began compressions, which I intermittently paused long enough for the anesthesiologist to deliver hand-forced ventilation. *Nothing.* Then the defibrillator paddles administered electric shocks immediately after the junior resident called, "Clear!" *No response.* According to protocol, adrenaline was administered via the IV. *Nothing.*

We continued this futile relay for at least 10 minutes.

Movies and fiction don't prepare you for the strange banality of watching a person die. The emotions on the moribund person's face are a combination of fear, helplessness, regret, and surprise. One moment the light is on, and then the next breath simply doesn't happen. Even though I knew I wasn't to blame, I still felt responsible.

I will never forget the sound of her ribs cracking under my compressions, the feculent fluid that spattered from her mouth (or the Tourette's-like profanity that spewed from the anesthesiologist's), and how, when we finally called off our efforts, her body's final sound was a loud and horrid seven-second release of gas from above and below, owing to the ventilated air having entered her GI tract instead of her lungs.

Why would I subject you to such a vivid and grim tale of death?

As cringe-worthy as it is, this account is a fitting allegory of my medical profession's unspoken core values. Doctors orchestrate medications, tests, procedures, hospitalizations, and hospice care without doing anything to seek a transformation of a desperate situation into a more hopeful one. In the vast majority of cases, doctors rarely try to prevent disease, they don't question the standard of care, and, most importantly, they don't offer hope, because deep down, they wrongly believe that life is inexorably meant to be a futile march toward death.

Your entire life, hopefully, won't disintegrate in two hours on a gurney. But chances are that your health and vitality *will* deteriorate over the last two decades of your life. If you don't die suddenly, then I can virtually guarantee you that your chart will be adorned with ultimately pointless lab testing, radiographs, MRIs, CAT scans, video explorations into various orifices, and an increasing number of prescriptions to manage whatever conditions with which you are tagged. You're likely to see multiple physicians and specialists, who will add their own feckless potions and regimens to your ever-expanding and "buffed" chart.

That unfortunate lady had a zero percent chance of survival without emergency reoperation, and probably less than a 10 percent chance of making it out of the hospital even if she did go back under the knife. Knowing the slim odds, the doctor and residents quite *ethically* chose to forgo extreme measures that would entail much suffering and instead to "buff her chart." But I'm here to tell you that the rest of your life doesn't have to be a short and quick (or long and slow) death march to this maudlin theme. You can march to a different beat.

Most doctors won't tell you this. As you approach your advancing state of physical and functional chaos, your medical professionals, possessed of the ethos of futility, would never suggest the possibility that aging and disease could ever be thwarted. Because of ignorance surrounding telomere biology, the notion that you might be saved from dying is anathema to the way doctors are trained to conceptualize aging. Growing old is dogmatically accepted as part of life's trajectory—it's normal. At least that is what we are told. But it isn't true.

It's time to flip the script.

WHY SHOULD YOU CARE ABOUT TELOMERES?

What if I'm right and there aren't a thousand diseases that can afflict us—there is only one disease with a thousand faces? Nearly all diseases can be understood as specific instances of one general principle at work: telomeres shorten in stem cells, causing genetic mutation—and *that* is why you should care about them. I've already mentioned a way to prevent the deterioration of health and function: telomerase. This enzyme is the basis of stem cell viability for all plants and animals on earth. So, telomeres and telomerase are the alpha and omega when it comes to aging and health. Still, most people (including most doctors and scientists) haven't yet grasped that all disease and aging share the same root cause.

Too simple to be true? I don't think so. I've witnessed miraculous improvements in telomere length associated with better sleep quality and quantity, more energy, improved appearance, better mood, and more efficient cellular repair and healing. I've experienced these benefits in myself, and I've helped thousands of people who have trusted my philosophy to enjoy more active, healthier, and "younger" living.

How you practice these age-defying strategies and incorporate them into your life is what this book is all about. My philosophy and practices are based on my own experience with countless patients and a wealth of research available to us all—but my passion for the science of telomeres was born from a highly personal wake-up call.

IT ALL HITS HOME

Even though I have witnessed death as a doctor, it truly wasn't until 2004 (when I was 37 years old) that the threat of aging, disease, and death hit home, literally. That was the year my father was diagnosed with brain cancer. Never sick a day in his life, the original "Dr. Park" was also a medical doctor, so when the brain tumor was discovered, he understood full well the horrors of what lay before him. He entertained the idea of refusing all treatments, but as anyone who has experienced a terminal diagnosis will explain, the tendency, even for a medical professional, is to believe that maybe *you* will defy the odds and be the exception to the rule. Perhaps even more ghastly, I suspect that Dad, like many patients, felt obliged to try something, for his family's sake and despite the suffering to come.

This vibrant man's swift decline under standard medical care is what sparked my interest in understanding why we grow old and infirm. As I watched my father deteriorate, something quietly shifted inside my core, and I knew at a deep level that I would try to find a way to help eradicate the pain, disease, and suffering that accompany aging and dying as we know it.

I was there the night he died at home, with his loved ones by his side. He had lost his ability to speak or move, and breathing had become a struggle. Despite that, he was still conscious and aware, like a shut-in. I could see the fear in his eyes, and just as I had with the Crohn's patient, I held his hand, reassured him, and watched him take his last breath. Months earlier, my father had talked of wanting to end his life. Given the quality of his last 12 months of existence—aggressive chemotherapy, radiation, cancer growing throughout his brain, and all the pain and suffering that comes from such treatments and disease—I was certain that he welcomed his release from the suffering.

While I came to terms with the difficult truth that I couldn't save my dad from terminal cancer, I was determined to find answers that would help my family, friends, patients, and myself.

I started by investigating and questioning all the available scientific information, research, and ideas about aging, and that led me to research that suggested an alternative to the inevitability of growing old. When I've got questions on my mind, I'm the sort of person who *relentlessly* asks "Why?" until I run out of questions. This characteristic of having an open mind, coupled with access to the vast knowledge available via the Internet, lends itself to learning just about anything in a relatively short amount of time—and that's just what I did.

This book is the result of what began as a personal mission to understand my father's illness and became a calling to share with the world this great news: *we already possess the capacity to turn back time in our bodies.*

WHY BELIEVE ME?

I've got the medical and scientific background you can trust, but I have zero interest in being the next guru of health. My passion derives from the results I see in the hundreds of patients I work with regularly. These are good people who are looking for better answers in their own personal journeys to halt the aging process. I simply want to open your mind to the alternate possibilities and a better way of growing older without growing old, by lengthening your telomeres through lifestyle choices.

I've written this book to organize and clearly present the scientific research as it relates to telomeres and then use that knowledge to create an effective, sustainable, and enjoyable plan that will increase telomerase activity. I hope that this will result in improved health and energy, a stronger immune system, a lower risk of disease, and an increased healthy and productive life for you.

Many of the popular theories and science on aging that I investigated seemed fanciful and absurd. It wasn't until I learned about telomeres and telomerase that my intuition was sparked. As I looked more deeply into the most popular theories on aging, only the telomere connection resonated, and that still holds true today.

This isn't just one man's fringe thinking.

A Few Examples of Telomere Science

Billions of dollars are spent each year to fund research around the impact of telomeres and telomerase on health. The result is currently more than 20,000 published studies, most of which establish an undeniable relationship between preserved telomeres, better health, and lower disease incidence—and longer lives. To the detriment of us all, researchers rarely consider the specific diseases as part of a universal process, as I do. Consider the following sampling of just a few of the thousands of scientific papers available to us:

- **Short telomeres = short lives.** In an ongoing study funded by the National Institutes of Health, researchers found that of more than 100,000 adults age 65 and older, those with the shortest telomere length had a more than 20 percent greater risk of dying in the following three years than those with longer telomeres. Beginning in 2009, the joint research team from the University of California–San Francisco and Kaiser Permanente collected yearly DNA samples from saliva to determine telomere length, and after five years, it determined a consistent elevated risk of mortality among those who had the shortest telomeres. The researchers also found that the more alcohol consumption and smoking increased, the shorter the telomeres were.[2]

- **Reduced heart disease.** Researchers at the University of Utah found that among people older than 60, those with shorter telomeres were three times more likely to die from heart disease and eight times more likely to die from infectious diseases than those with longer telomeres. The study tracked 143 unrelated Utah residents, ages 60 to 97, whose telomere length was measured from blood tests from 1982 to 1986; at the study's conclusion, 101 of the adults had died. The researchers found that when taking the question of mortality as a whole, those with longer telomeres live on average five years longer than those with shorter telomeres. The researchers speculate that the increase in life span could be from 10 to 30 years.[3]

- **Postmortem proof.** Researchers at the University of Washington evaluated telomere length in more than 1,000 adults. Upon learning of a participant's death, they compared medical records and telomere lengths to the cause of death. Deaths from infectious causes were 280 percent higher and death from heart disease was 60 percent more likely in those with the shortest telomeres.[4]

- **Live longer.** A Danish study published in 2015 that tracked more than 64,000 people over seven years found that longer telomeres were associated with longer life spans. The researchers found that those who had longer telomeres also had lower blood pressure and LDL cholesterol compared to those with shorter telomeres.[5]

- **Eat right to live longer.** In the largest study ever to assess the association between telomere length and adherence to a Mediterranean diet, researchers from Harvard Medical School found that of more than 4,600 women ages 42 to 70, those who ate Mediterranean diets had significantly longer telomeres than those who didn't. This style of diet is defined as being rich in vegetables, fruits, nuts, whole grains, legumes, fish, and olive oil and has been connected to lower rates of heart disease, cancer, inflammation, high blood pressure, and obesity in many other published studies. The 2014 study, published in the *British Medical Journal*, tested blood samples to determine telomere length and compared this to detailed diet questionnaires that the women completed.[6]

- **Move more for longer telomeres.** Sedentary behavior increases your risk of having shorter telomeres, according to Swedish researchers. The six-month long study, published in the *British Journal of Sports Medicine*, consisted of 49 adults, 68 years old, who were sedentary and overweight. The men and women were randomly assigned to either an intervention group, which encouraged an increase in steps per day and a decrease in time spent sitting, or a control group that didn't receive any activity-related advice. Blood samples were collected at the beginning and end of the six-month trial to determine telomere length. In addition to decreases in weight, fat, and cholesterol, the group that moved more and sat less increased their telomeres significantly, while those who remained sedentary had shorter telomeres.[7]

- **Sleep for a longer life.** According to Robert Wood Johnson Foundation researchers, poor sleep quality equals shorter telomeres. The study, published in the *Journal of Aging Research*, evaluated the average nightly sleep quality of 245 women, ages 49 to 66, against their telomere length (determined from blood samples). The investigators found that women who reported difficulty falling asleep, restless sleep, and early waking all had shorter telomeres than those who reported good sleep quality.[8]

YOU'RE NEVER TOO OLD TO GET YOUNGER (AND NEVER TOO YOUNG TO GET OLDER)

You may be thinking, "At what point is it too late to turn back time?" The short answer is: never. You're never too old to get younger. The flip side of this is that you're never too young to get older either. The premature aging of progeria that we discussed earlier proves that chronological age isn't what matters, it's cellular aging from genetic damage. Considering only telomere lengths, you actually "aged" most rapidly from the time you were conceived up until the moment you were born. You actually burned through one-third of your telomeres *in utero*. It is possible that some cellular aging is needed for fetal development and normal puberty, but once you are fully developed as a young adult, you can safely slow the aging process by activating telomerase. What if diseases are simply the result of faulty cells? If we destroy the faulty stem cells and replace them, we can reverse the diseases. Unfortunately, medicine views most diseases as permanent conditions rather than temporary aberrations, and the orthodox treatments usually involve some drug that further blocks or alters normal functioning.

Nobody would buy a new car and then neglect oil changes and regular maintenance until it broke down, right? My point is that taking much better care of your body *before* it breaks down is a better strategy. What if we treated our bodies like priceless vintage cars—regardless of previous maintenance and repair history? There are truly powerful actions you can take to slow and even stop the progression of aging as we know it, and this book will introduce them to you.

SPOILER ALERT: I am going to come clean and just let you peer behind the Wizard of Oz's curtain now: most of what I present in *The Telomere Miracle* will seem like common sense, like *get enough sleep* and *exercise regularly*. So why even read it? Because you will build a deep and unshakable understanding of your physiology, and because the research based on telomere research will point toward the best practices for harnessing your body's natural rejuvenating power.

Everywhere, we are told to welcome the deterioration of health until an inevitable costly and fruitless final stand, either in an ICU or in an old-folks' home (nearly 70 percent of Americans die in a hospital or a nursing home[9]). The other 30 percent? Well, hopefully, like my father, many people will be at home with loved ones close by when they pass. Still, my father's suffering was too great to justify the futile and rather barbaric treatments that he received. I have come to believe that there's a better way, because I have seen it in the people I work with every day.

I have attended thousands of fetal births as an ob-gyn, but the "rebirths" are more poignant, because older adults recognize how precious life is. Instead of driving through the night to usher a confused baby into the world, my practice affords me the opportunity to share e-mails and phone calls from patients in their 70s and 80s who have decided there is time enough and passion enough to start a new career or romantic relationship or master a new skill. These are the people who have shifted their perspective and believe that growing old and deteriorating is not inevitable. This cosmic U-turn that indicates *these people are no longer winding down or counting the days until life is over—they can see that aging is optional.*

Studies indicate that aging, as measured by newborns' telomere length, is accelerated even in utero when the mother is stressed or obese. So, aging can start even before your first breath. On the other hand, research also shows that relaxation techniques can slow the shortening of telomeres—which slows your aging.

There is nothing qualitatively different about normal cellular rejuvenation or deterioration in your advanced years; you have just accumulated a lot more of it.

A SUDDEN TRANSFORMATION

About a year into my research on telomeres and aging, I was introduced to a supplement that was shown to increase telomerase activity and to protect and preserve telomeres. I was skeptical, but the scientists who isolated the natural molecule provided me with enough research on its safety and efficacy that I decided to give it a try. Within a short time, my body began to transform. Without changing my diet or adding exercise, I lost 15 pounds, my sleep improved drastically, and my friends and patients began to take notice of my weight loss and increased energy. When they insisted that I share my "secret," I became the first physician to practice what I call "telomerase activation medicine," and I have been successful in helping many thousands of people find their own paths back to better health and wellness. Since that time, many other doctors have prescribed similar supplements to help people reverse aging. By combining my knowledge of this supplement with other research-supported lifestyle strategies, I've been able to help many patients to enhance telomerase activity and to restore their telomeres.

HARNESSING THE POWER OF TELOMERES

Imagine you're illiterate. You speak your native language fluently, but you can't read or write. You likely have some understanding of how language and speech work, but you lack the full picture that comes from understanding the complexities of grammar, punctuation, vocabulary, communication, and more that comprehending written language would give you. In other words, by becoming more educated, you gain a deeper and more intricate understanding of something you already know (in this case, verbal language).

Similarly, you might not be a health expert, but you already are an expert regarding what it takes to stay healthier for longer. This knowledge includes things such as avoiding overeating, getting exercise, sleeping well, and being happy. However, you, like most of the population, probably don't do those things as well as you *could*, because you don't fully appreciate how these behaviors actually help your body to repair and prevent aging.

So . . .

The Telomere Miracle is going to introduce you to scientific evidence and simple theories so that you will be Ph.D.-level literate in the language of health and longevity. The techniques you will learn are no mystery, but deeper self-study will lead to an intuitive and profound understanding of how the TeloMirror tools can help you delay aging and disease. What you eventually do with the knowledge you acquire from this book will depend on your ability to trust your intuition and not just rely on experts who regurgitate groupthink.

There are other books on telomeres, but this book aims to marry the science surrounding telomeres with personalized strategies that help enhance wellness from within. Your mission, should you choose to accept it, is simply to open your mind to the possibility that perhaps aging and disease are not as natural, predetermined, and inevitable as you once believed.

Ready? Let's get to it.

HOW TO USE THIS BOOK

If your idea of staying young and being healthy means self-deprivation and a morbid sense of guilt, then you should probably put down this book and walk away.

I'm more of a go-with-the-flow type. If that sounds more enjoyable, then take a slow deep breath in and then exhale. That's how easy it is to get your body on board with preserving your telomeres and rejuvenating your cells. To paraphrase Glinda the Good Witch's words of wisdom to Dorothy in *The Wizard of Oz*: you've always had the power inside; you just need to learn how to access it. So stop worrying, because it really isn't helping. Even in the face of uncertainty, fear, and perceived scarcity, let us persevere with humor, love, and generosity. Living in a constant state of paranoia, worry, and self-deprivation, even with the intention of achieving optimal health, is a life poorly lived and probably makes matters worse in the grand scheme of things.

We've already covered a lot of ground in this chapter. You now know what telomeres are, that telomerase keeps them long in stem cells, and why we should harness telomerase to prevent aging and illness. Chapters 2 and 3 will complete your foundational knowledge of all you need to grasp the fundamentals of this new Unified Stem Cell Telomere Theory. You'll learn strategies that will heal your body at a cellular level to provide overall balance and health in your body.

In Part II, Chapters 4 through 9, we'll cover six cylinders that will power the engine of your optimal life. These six *TeloMirror Tools* (TMTs) are your breath, mind, sleep, exercise, nutrition, and supplements. You will learn how each of these systems works and why they tend to deteriorate with age. In those chapters, your belief in my theory will grow stronger as we look at the research proving how those systems can be either helping or hurting your telomere integrity and therefore your overall health. After all, we are made up entirely of cells and those cells all obey the same rules. One disease, six cylinders, and a thousand ways to deteriorate if we are passive or ignorant of the power we possess.

Part III is where you will integrate these new habits into your life. In Chapter 10 you'll get your quick-start guide to all the self-assessment and prep work you need for a full toolbox of TMTs, which will keep you moving toward your anti-aging goals. In Chapter 11, you'll learn how to continue to track your daily, weekly, and monthly habits to preserve your telomeres and live a happier, healthier, and longer life. Finally, in Chapter 12, I will outline exciting future developments that I believe may bring about the absolute end of aging itself. Someday, as a result of bioengineering, common sense, and self-mastery, we can anticipate getting older without significantly aging as we currently understand it.

MY VISION FOR YOU

By reading this book, you will gain insight on how to master your breathing, thoughts, sleep, exercise, nutrition, and supplements. These are the six cylinders that drive the engine of a healthy life, and my goal is to get you firing on all cylinders.

This book is my attempt to organize and clearly present the scientific research as it is being reflected in our "TeloMirrors" and to then offer an effective, sustainable, and enjoyable plan that will preserve your telomeres by increasing telomerase activity. All this will hopefully enable improved health and energy, a stronger immune system, a lower rate of disease, and an increased healthy and productive life span. With this in mind, I hope you'll:

- Learn a new paradigm of aging that allows for the possibility of growing younger and more vibrant as the years pass

- Be inspired by the scientific research to continue learning

- Improve your life from the inside out with continuous self-assessment and improvement of your six areas of TeloMirror *maintenance*

- Abandon the experts who have abandoned all hope in favor of simply "buffing your chart"

Our goal is to live healthy, happy, and long lives—now you can. Welcome to the future of aging. You may have to give up some old ideas but I believe that the time you invest in reading will be returned to you many times over.

My best advice for living longer? Stop trying so hard, and read on.

Chapter 2

Biology 101—
Genetics and Cell Biology

Truth is easy to grasp and hard to vary.

So, what are the essential facts you need to know about how your body—and, for that matter, how all living organisms on earth are organized and function? We aren't talking about your car, your computer, or something that might become obsolete. We are talking about the fundamentals of biology—and it is not reducible beyond a certain level of complexity. So, this chapter aims to fill you in on the essentials about the mechanics of your organism on a cellular level. I have tried to make the explanations that follow clear and simple—but not at the expense of The Ultimate Goal: to have you clearly understand how biology keeps us young and healthy, yet also enables you to grow old and infirm. To get the most from this chapter, consider my thoughts about the one cause of aging with an open mind. Although it may take a bit of learning and possibly some suspension of old beliefs, you will be changed, perhaps even transformed (in a positive way), by the implications.

Despite its many facets, all we think of as being associated with growing old, and most of the diseases that accompany it, can be explained by one root cause:

Aging is the result of DNA damage enabled by the telomere shortening that occurs in stem cells over time.

Below is my theory of aging in a nutshell. You probably won't be able to make much sense of this right now—and that's okay. By the end of the chapter you might just be an expert.

My Telomere and Stem Cell Theory of Aging

- Axiom 1:
  Telomeres always shorten when one cell divides into two, and when telomeres become critically short, the cell malfunctions and/or dies from resulting chromosome mutation.

- Axiom 2:
  Non-stem cells cannot reproduce indefinitely.

- Axiom 3:
  A daughter cell can only be as healthy (genetic integrity) or as young (telomere length) as the stem cell it came from.

- Axiom 4:
  Stem cells can restore telomere length with telomerase (I explain Axiom 4 further later in this chapter).

- Hypothesis:
  Aging is caused by the shortening of telomeres in stem cells. Therefore, if telomerase activity increases in stem cells, then telomere length will be preserved and the effects of aging will be slowed and possibly reversed.

But let's back up for a minute. Before we return to my theory, I want us all on the same page with respect to genetics and cells. To understand how this whole telomere/aging thing works, you need to have some basic knowledge about the inner workings of your cells, the chromosomes inside those cells, on down to the telomeres on the ends of your chromosomes. Don't worry, there won't be any quizzes, and the following bit of adult education is meant to be enriching and even interesting. Whatever soaks in, great—you don't need to fully assimilate all the information—but do try to get the gist of what I'm saying.

Let's get to it.

CHROMOSOMES, DNA, AND GENES

As you probably know, our body is mainly made up of organs, connective tissue, and blood. Cells are membrane-surrounded actors responsible for making up those organs, producing the connective tissue, and giving rise to blood. Inside every one of our trillions of cells is a smaller bubble inside the larger cell that we call the nucleus. The cell's nucleus houses your chromosomes, which are tightly twisted-up bundles of DNA and can be thought of as two redundant 23-volume cookbook sets that make up a 46-volume set that contains all the required genetic information for creating and operating you.

Twenty-three chromosomes came from your mom's egg, and the other 23 came from your dad's sperm. If a cell is going to divide, it makes duplicates of all 46, still connected at the centromeres like Siamese twins that look like bow-tie X's. Moments later, the 46 Siamese twins will become 46 single chromosomes in one cell and 46 single and identical chromosomes in the other.

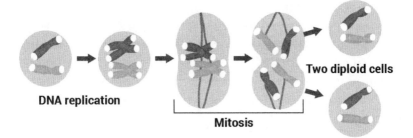

DNA replication

Two diploid cells

Mitosis

When we are young and healthy, the chromosomes in every cell are nearly identical; as we age, we tend to accumulate damaged chromosomes with incorrect numbers. That is why we start to show signs of aging and dysfunction.

If Chromosomes and DNA Are the Same, Why Are They Referred To by Two Different Names?

Chromosomes are made up of end-to-end, complementary, matched and twisted pairs of DNA chains that are spooled around proteins called histones. Each chromosome is like a single discrete cookbook measuring about 50,000,000 to 250,000,000 base pairs (see below) and each contains from 200 to 2,000 genes, which are DNA sequences that specify the recipes for each of our 20,000 unique proteins.

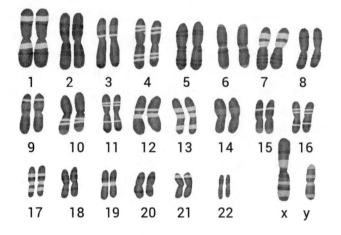

The genes in the vast majority of healthy human beings are encoded identically and located in precisely the same spot on the same chromosome, because we are all closely related. In contrast, nearly identical genes can be scattered among different numbers of chromosomes if two species are not closely related. There is a semiaquatic rodent from Venezuela that has 92 chromosomes, for example.

Chromosomes are numbered by decreasing size, so Mom's egg gave you her biggest Chromosome 1 and Dad's sperm also gave you his biggest Chromosome 1. The 23rd pair are the so-called sex chromosomes, so if you are a man, you got one X chromosome (the name, not the shape) from Mom and a Y chromosome from Dad. If you are a woman, you got an X chromosome from Mom and another X chromosome from Dad. Remember progeria and the effects of only getting one functioning telomerase gene? Luckily, most of the time all the chromosomes that we inherit have both maternal and paternal working copies of all our genes.

Much of the time, a chromosome looks like a sausage with a tight belt at the center body, or centromere. The X or bow-tie appearance only occurs when a cell is getting ready to divide into two cells, like Siamese twins about to be surgically separated.

For most of a cell's life, its chromosomes are actually partially unpacked, like spaghetti in a pot of boiling water. Your chromosomes are relaxed so that your micromachines can easily access and transcribe the genes in the DNA (more on this later).

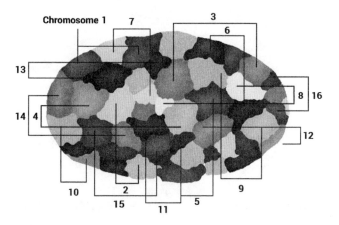

Some cells never divide, but those that do will gather all bow-tie Siamese twins and then tear them apart. This is the critical moment when the havoc caused by telomere erosion, namely fused double chromosomes, comes home to roost. When you try to give 46 copies to one daughter cell and 46 to the other but some of the chromosomes are fused together, you will have damaged sets of cookbooks in both daughter cells.

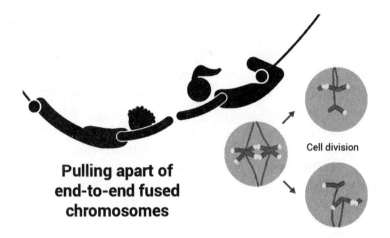

Pulling apart of end-to-end fused chromosomes

Cell division

Think of fused chromosomes as trapeze artists with hands irreversibly sewn together. Now make the trapeze infinitely stronger than the force of gravity. What transpires is that one side of the circus gets two trapeze artists, or gets a torn-up and bloody artist with some extra arms or half a torso whereas the other side of the circus gets just a trunk and legs.

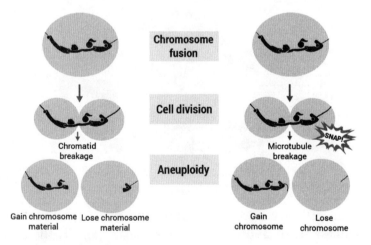

Chromosome fusion

Cell division

Chromatid breakage

SNAP!

Microtubule breakage

Aneuploidy

Gain chromosome material Lose chromosome material

Gain chromosome Lose chromosome

If the "ropes" (really microtubules) pulling the chromosomes apart break before the fused chromosomes, you will get a different problem of uneven segregation. One daughter gets both trapeze artists and the other gets none. This aneuploidy (from the Greek for "not right number") not only drives things like Down syndrome, it is the final common destiny of every cell that survives long enough to undergo telomere-associated mutation.

So, What Is DNA and What Are Genes?

DNA is the information-storage method used for all living things. (NOTE: There are rare viruses and even proteins that present exceptions to the rule of DNA-based life, but all the other viruses, bacteria, and living things use DNA.) DNA is a single molecule that assembles into polymer chains, which are also called DNA even if they are a million single units long. The four flavors of DNA: adenine (A), guanine (G), cytosine (C), and thymine (T). DNA rules of bonding say that adenine (A) is always paired across the helix with thymine (T); guanine (G) is always paired across the helix with cytosine (C). So, along your DNA double helix, it looks like this:

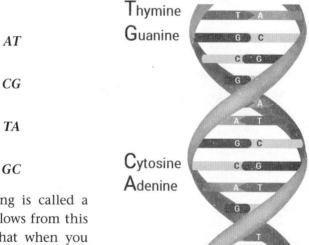

Thymine

Guanine

AT

CG

TA

GC

Cytosine
Adenine

Each pairing is called a *base pair.* It follows from this pairing rule that when you know that one portion of a single strand of DNA code reads "ATGCAA," then the only way to form the double helix, or stable rope ladder, is to have the other matching single strand of DNA read "TACGTT." Do you get it? The complementary matching system means each side serves as a template for its perfect mate.

If you had a mass-produced death mask mold of Julius Caesar's face, you could create the positive clay statue from the mold or, conversely, create another negative mold from the statue.

The paired strands not only provide for a redundant information storage method, they also provide protection from damage. Imagine if a ladder were cut into two halves, vertically; those halves would be less stable and easier to alter than a whole ladder where each rung reinforces the overall structure.

The order in which the base pairs occur, like the words in a cookbook, determine the recipes that direct how unique proteins are to be assembled. Proteins are also chains, but they are single strands made up of amino acids. The order of their assembly is what is encoded by sequences of DNA in the genes. Thanks to DNA-sequencing technology, scientists have deduced what some DNA sequence changes confer in terms of rare diseases and other traits, but we still have a lot to learn. Amazingly, this four-letter alphabet, comprising just those four "letters," determines your genes, and that is why scientists refer to your complete set of genes in your 46 chromosomes as your **genome**.

To recap: Every cell's nucleus has a complete set of 23 Mom and 23 Pop chromosomes, made from DNA, which are like cookbooks for the genes that will be transcribed and then translated into proteins that magically assemble into cells and the rest of you. You inherit your genes from your parents and their ancestors. Genes are discrete recipes with specific locations on specific chromosomes. As we will understand more clearly soon, critically short telomeres produce fused chromosomes, which lead to chromosomal chaos in future cell descendants, such as breaks, duplications, and absences of the perfect 46 matched sets we were given at birth. The illustration on page 31 is a depiction of this process, at the heart of all cell dysfunction and death, as a form of "genetic entropy" known as chromothripsis.

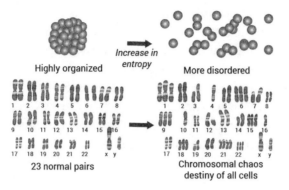

Highly organized → *Increase in entropy* → More disordered

23 normal pairs

Chromosomal chaos destiny of all cells

You may choose to take what I just said on faith. If not, you can easily grasp every step of the science behind it by simply reading on.

DNA Replication: The Engine of Aging

In the first sense, copying DNA drives aging because it is what tech people would call a slightly "lossy" process. Every time a cell divides, an average of 0.32 typographical errors are made, which is pretty darn good for 3.2 billion letters in the old 46-volume cookbook.

A more punctuated and cataclysmic driver of aging by chromosomal mutation occurs when telomeres become critically short. This is driven by two simple truths of DNA replication: directionality of assembly and the so-called "end replication problem."

1. One half of each helix, or the 3'→5' (read as "three prime to five prime") strand, is the antisense or leading strand. It is called antisense because it is an inverse, like Caesar's death mask, which is transcribed into the message RNA TRANSCRIPT (Caesar's positive facial image, which will be TRANSLATED into a protein; more on this later). It is called "leading" because its matching, complementary strand can and will be assembled, literally seamlessly, in the 5'→3' direction. These numbers refer to the carbon numbers in the DNA sugar molecules.

2. The 5'→3' strand, or lagging strand, is copied by splicing together of segments called "Okazaki fragments" (named for the scientist who discovered them). On the complementary strand made from matching this strand, you will require seams. The lagging strand runs in a 5'→3' direction, so its complementary 3'→5' strand can't be assembled continuously. That means the process lags, or is slower, on this half of the unzipped helix. In all life everywhere (except in bacteria with circular DNA), a temporary RNA primer must be laid down allowing for discontinuous 5'→3' segments, or Okazaki fragments, to be made. The segments are spliced together at these primer "seams." Then the RNA primer sequences are replaced with regular DNA. Since there is no way to attach the primer to the very tip of the lagging strand during replication (or even within 50 to 100 base pairs of the ends of the telomere), we encounter what scientists call the end-replication problem.

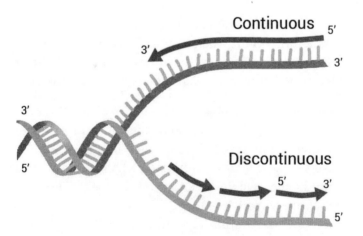

This end-replication "problem" is what drives *replicative senescence*, a term that refers to the fact that most cells cannot divide indefinitely. As the term implies, telomerase-inactive cell lines will naturally "get older from copying." This loss of a little blank tape with each copying is the reason non-stem cells will encounter the Hayflick limit (again, named for the scientist who documented it), which refers to the 50 to 70 possible divisions of a cell's descendants before non-viability (cell death).

HAYFLICK LIMIT

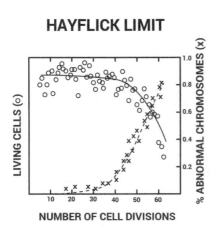

NUMBER OF CELL DIVISIONS

But there isn't any reason to panic; it's all part of a grand plan. In fact, the term *end replication problem* is misleading. You wouldn't call the loss of leaves from a maple tree the wasted leaves problem, right? Like leaves, many of your cells are meant to lose telomeres in their DNA and die off so they can be replaced by newer, healthier cells, more recently derived from model stem cells. The planned obsolescence of non-stem cells caused by replicative senescence and the Hayflick limit is normal, and the system is more concerned with the preservation and integrity of model stem cells.

With replicative senescence in stem cells, the stakes are higher. If a bit of telomere length is lost every time your DNA is copied and the cell divides, and it is not restored by telomerase, at some point a critical amount of telomere length is depleted, and then something very bad happens. Without blank-tape telomeres, the cell-repair machinery misinterprets the uncapped end as a double strand break and uses a splicing enzyme to splice the end of one chromosome to the end of another, producing a fused, double chromosome. This "double strand breakage repair" is an ancient and essential process, and it is a very good thing, because sometimes DNA does come apart and needs to be quickly spliced or glued back together. But if normally discrete chromosomes becomes fused at the ends in a stem cell, the next time that stem cell divides, there will be no way for both of the resulting cells to get a perfect number of chromosomes. Instead, chromosomes will be torn apart or divided unevenly between the two daughters.

If you want to talk about a real "problem," that would be when telomere ends erode and cause mutations of chromosomes in your immortal stem cells. Once a nonlethal change is introduced into these model cells, it is hard to get rid of, because stem cells relengthen telomeres and live on indefinitely. Now we have a problem, because instead of expendable leaves, we have bad stems (pun intended) that are producing damaged leaves. Experiments in mice suggest that a good way to combat aging is to actually enhance damaged cells' abilities to kill themselves in processes known as apoptosis (cell death) and autophagy (self-consumption).[1]

That is the reason stem cell damage from telomere erosion is so dangerous. Run-of-the-mill leaves can die. Bad immortal stems might not be as easy to kill off, and they start producing bad cells, which make poorly functioning and aging organs. If you don't think this is a real problem, consider that nearly all cancer cell lines display exactly these kinds of chromosomal fusions and duplications, which can best be attributed to replicative senescence of telomeres, leading to end-to-end fusions and producing aneuploid ("not right number") cells after mitosis. So all of aging and disease could actually be a result of the accumulation of nonlethal mutations in stem cell chromosomes throughout our body as well as the slow depletion of the reserves of stem cells in our bone marrow.

Now let's delve deeper into how your chromosomes' genes actually make proteins. Remember, when we start chopping up chromosomes and duplicating or eliminating gene copies, we are losing important recipes for enzymes that protect, monitor, and regulate our cells.

The Central Dogma of Molecular Biology is gene *transcription* into messenger ribonucleic acid (mRNA) and mRNA *translation* into proteins. This is how the antisense gene recipe is written into a sense mRNA message, which is then sent to the protein assembly factory called the ribosomes (the short-order cook).

Although it must be more complex in ways we can't yet imagine, at this moment, science believes that all the things we are come simply from the production of proteins.[2] Proteins are long chains of molecules, called amino acids, that are assembled like beads on a string and then fold up like origami micromachines. Cell function, or dysfunction, depends on having the correct proteins made. Cells need to constantly assemble and update their proteins for optimal structure and function. And for the most part, the proteins are for use only inside their cells of origin.

There's still more to how we actually make the proteins. Remember, your genes contain the instructions but they must be transcribed into a message—that's where messenger RNA comes into play. RNA is very similar to DNA, but the RNA has an extra oxygen in a place that the deoxy (no oxygen) DNA does not. This allows RNA to travel around as a water-soluble single strand.

There are other flavors of RNA, but right now, let's stick to discussing mRNA, whose principal role is to carry the transcribed gene recipe out of the nucleus to the cytoplasm (the space outside the inner nucleus but still inside the cell membrane). In the cytoplasm, protein-building machines will translate the mRNA into proteins that create you. Here's how it all works:

When new proteins are needed in the cell, an enzyme in the nucleus known as RNA polymerase ("-ase" means enzyme and "polymer" means a molecule made up of many units) will attach to the start of the unzipped antisense 3'→5' antisense gene that is the negative image of the instructions for the type of protein needed. Like DNA, RNA is assembled in the 5'→3' direction. The RNA polymerase moves along the DNA strand and synthesizes a single strand mRNA. This process is called gene *transcription.*

Then, like a waiter tearing off a ticket in a diner, the mRNA order is sent to the short-order cook known as the ribosomes. mRNA moves out of the nucleus and into the cytoplasm of a cell, where there those ribosomes transcribe the mRNA instructions into an actual protein, one amino acid at a time. These amino acids fold into the three-dimensional shape and type of protein needed. Proteins are made up of amino acids, and there are a total of 20 different flavors of amino acids. The order and type of amino acids in a protein chain determine how the protein will take shape and what function it will serve—there are many. Proteins can be part of your immune system, such as antibodies; they can serve as enzymes; they are signaling hormones like insulin; they are part of muscle fibers; they transport oxygen; and much more. Suffice it to say that proteins do most of the work in our bodies.

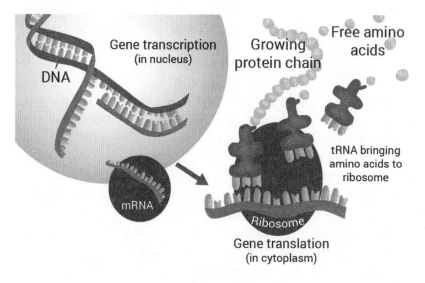

This process of building proteins happens in the same way in all living organisms. You may not find that useful or interesting, but biologists are pretty happy to know that the same exact mechanisms for creating proteins and functioning cells are the same for the *bacteria* living in the stomach of the *insect* feeding on the *tree* that made the paper of the book *you* are reading. There is no other way to make proteins for use in cells—this master recipe is the same for all life—and that is why it's called The Central Dogma of Molecular Biology.

Different genes are turned "on" (to be made into different proteins) and "off" at any given time in different types of cells for different reasons. The genes being expressed are the genes that are "on," and this is referred to as gene expression. Remember, every cell in your body received two sets of cookbooks (23 from Mom,

23 from Dad), which means that all your cells could express all 20,000 or more genes that are encoded in your DNA at any given time, but they don't, because that would be chaos. It needs to be this way so that our genes can all have specialized cells that provide organized functions, so that our complex human organism can work properly. Liver cells need to act and function like proper liver cells to detoxify, heart cells must act and function like heart cells so blood can be pumped to all your body parts, and so on. The genes a cell expresses determine what kind of restaurant the cell will be.

> *To sum up where we are now: DNA contains the information, but it needs mRNA to transcribe the information and then carry it out of the nucleus, where it can be translated by protein-building machines that can then manufacture the actual chains of amino acids that make up proteins. Easy, right?*

STEM CELLS—THE SECRET OF IMMORTALITY

We have already discussed cells, how they divide, and how they contain DNA, genes, proteins, and so on. Now we need to discuss the difference between your regular cells and your stem cells. There are about 200 types of cells that make up the trillions of cells that make up the human body—liver cells, skin cells, hair cells, stomach cells, bone cells, brain cells, and so on. These are what we call *differentiated cells*, meaning they have specific jobs that require specialized gene expression set forth by their epigenetic software applications (to be discussed later). A liver cell doesn't wake up one day and decide to be a bone cell. When a liver cell divides and replicates, it can only become liver cells, just as bone cells become bone cells, and so on. That is because of differentiation of stem cells that began way back when you were an itty-bitty fetus.

The Genesis

You, me, and everyone you know originated from one single stem cell: the zygote (or fertilized egg). This one cell is quite literally the mother of all stem cells, because it has the innate ability to become all the cells that create you. You probably remember the movie shown back in your school's health class of the little fertilized egg dividing and becoming a mass of little balls. That first stem cell divided and divided, and eventually the differentiation and specialization begat your skin, hair, organs, and, well, you.

But that is not the end of your stem cells. These rather magical cells remain in all areas and organs of your body all throughout your life. They live, die, and are replaced over time. Your liver has liver stem cells, your brain has brain stem cells, your bones have stem cells, and so on. These adult stem cells are specialized to that organ's cell type and reign over their own tiny kingdoms, or *stem cell niches*.

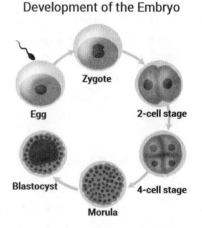

Development of the Embryo

What Makes a Cell Stem-Like?

In general, there are two properties of stem-ness: *immortality* and *asymmetric division*. First, immortality in stem cells is facilitated by telomerase, the enzyme that adds back telomeres to reverse replicative senescence, keeping that stem cell alive indefinitely (in the last section of this chapter I'll explain the details of how telomerase works). Asymmetric division means that a stem cell can make one perfect copy of herself, the immortal queen mother, but she also splits into specialized and differentiated daughters (regular mortal cells), which lack the capacity to use telomerase.

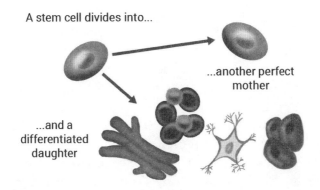

A stem cell divides into...

...another perfect mother

...and a differentiated daughter

So, the regular cells created by stem cells (also called differentiated daughter cells) go on to live regular cell lives. They divide to make regular cells and are subject to replicative senescence and the Hayflick limit. Let's say we are talking about your liver. These differentiated daughter cells (e.g., liver cells) can arise from another non-stem liver cell dividing in two, but they can also arise from the local liver *queen stem cell* that replenishes the cells for that niche. The more recently a cell had its origination from a queen (stem cell), the better its genetic integrity (the healthier and younger it is) and the longer its telomeres, unless that queen happens to be damaged or old.

Each queen (adult stem cell) *niche* is like a bee colony in which all daughters are clones of the mama queen—although if you were paying attention during the last paragraph, not all cells will be as perfect or as young as the hardworking queen. Scientists believe that your organs are composed of many queens and many niches, and so your entire liver is not made up of just one cell type but could have experienced some genetic variation over time based

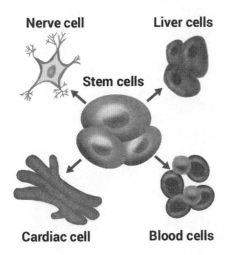

Nerve cell

Liver cells

Stem cells

Cardiac cell

Blood cells

on the regional niches and their queens' life histories and accumulated errors. If you drink a lot or have hepatitis, your liver stem cells have had to copy more than normal to replace diseased or dead cells, which means that these cells undergo more opportunities for introducing new errors from DNA copying and other vicissitudes of life.

In contrast, when a daughter cell comes from another daughter cell that was already 40 cell divisions removed from the original mama queen, that 41st generation of two differentiated daughters has a larger chance of inheriting errors and much shorter telomeres because of the 40 times its predecessors lived, suffered, and then copied their entire DNA library (*genome*).

The queen can keep herself immortal by using telomeres, unless she has acquired some gene mutations or aging; in that case, her daughters will inherit these as well and pass along the damage. The main mechanism of genetic errors in queen stem cells may be telomere shortening; however, there are other causes of cell damage, such as infectious agents, toxins, and radiation.

It is important to know that dysfunctional and soon-to-be-dead local and specialized queen stem cells (brain, heart, liver, and so on) have an external source of replacements. There is a master stem cell type, called *mesenchymal stem cells* (MSC), that can travel to all organs in search of niches with worn-out or dead queen stem cells in need of replacement. Those MSCs are less specialized and will undergo on-the-job training to take on the semi-permanent role of specialized queen bee wherever they end up settling down.

Apoptosis (Cell Suicide) Is a Good Thing

All cells have built-in, always-on systems that self-regulate, repair, or elicit suicide when they are damaged genetically. The emergent property of these trillions of cells with their programmed behaviors is that your body remains in a sustainable state of balance of creation, maintenance, and destruction for as long as it can. Telomere erosion and cell suicide from chromosomal mutation is fine for regular cells but is much more serious in stem cells, like having a mold of Caesar's face with errors: there is no chance that the statues the mold produces will be perfect anymore.

So, if stem cells are immortal, why don't they already keep us forever young? There are several issues:

First, telomerase can't always keep up with replicative senescence. DNA with shortened telomeres will fuse together and cause mutations. Maintaining telomere length in a cell is an active process, similar to walking up a 50-story escalator that is moving down.

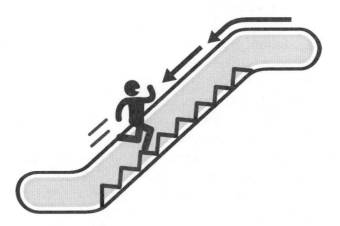

If you walk fast enough, with an equal and opposite tempo to the escalator's downward motion, you can stay at the same level. This represents cell division in which the telomeres are long enough to provide continued chromosome division and replication—everything stays healthy and equal, in balance. But if the moving stairs speed up beyond your capacity to walk fast enough, the escalator wins and you end up lower and lower until you find yourself in the basement. This is what happens when your cells are in a state of over-copying, as with the rapid turnover caused by damage and inflammation in an alcoholic's liver or a smoker's lungs. You may not be giving your system the time it needs to regain lost ground.

Second, errors and damage sometimes occur in the actual information contained on the chromosomal DNA (or genes) that resides between those shortening telomere caps. Here the genetic information gets damaged by transcription errors, viruses, radiation, and toxins, which causes irregularities in cell functioning because of gene mutation or functional deletion. If damaged yet immortalized stem cells reproduce, their dysfunction can manifest as diseases because all the cells from that queen's niche have the same genetic problems.

Third and most important, the available reserve of backup MSCs can become damaged and depleted over time from copying and from the introduction of typographical as well as environmentally produced errors. Stem cell depletion can be explained with this analogy: if you were born with a closet full of rechargeable batteries, eventually, because of the limited life spans of the rechargeable batteries being used, you would run out of unused, new rechargeable batteries in that storage closet.

This fact might explain what I call the "Redenbacher effect." When you're waiting for microwave popcorn, nothing seems to happen for a minute and a half and then it all starts to pop. Similarly, in our 70s or 80s we seem to encounter a crescendo of multiple problems at once. I used to think this synchrony was due to local stem cells in many organs failing at the same time, but perhaps it is due more to the common mesenchymal stem cell pool declining in quality and quantity from telomere shortening.

EPIGENETICS: WHY CELLS ARE DIFFERENT DESPITE HAVING THE SAME DNA

Science is still learning about other gene modifications, referred to as epigenetics, which means "outside the genes." If your various cellular organelles (mini-organs such as ribosomes, mitochondria, and so on) can be compared to a computer's hardware, then the genetic code of DNA would be the operating system, which is supposed to be nearly identical in all cells. Epigenetics would be like added software applications that help to aid and instruct your genes.

Epigenetic modifications to the DNA, by definition, don't alter the letter sequences per se, but instead dictate which proteins will be preferentially expressed and therefore what kind of behavior and appearance the cell will express. So instead of just buying a new computer and risking incorrectly reinstalling the software, a mother cell clones itself two identical clones and copies the same epigenetic software. We don't yet understand how this works.

In the case of an asymmetrically dividing queen stem cell, the queen copies the royal epigenetics and the better organelles to one future-mother daughter and also copies similar but slightly different epigenetic software to the other daughter. The reason we need to understand epigenetics is because it explains how certain cells specialize. The epigenetic software is there to make sure the cell expresses certain proteins and behaviors over others (including stemness) and accounts for why a liver stem cell and its liver daughters don't act like bone stem cells and their bone daughters.

GENETIC DAMAGE AND SIGNS OF AGING

A 19th-century Augustinian Czech monk, Gregor Mendel, is famous for doing experiments involving interbreeding beans, which uncovered many interesting principles that relate to the inheritance of traits. That is why clinical genetics and the way genes are inherited through sexual reproduction is now referred to as Mendelian genetics. The interesting and oft-ignored aspect of Mendelian genetics that is helpful for understanding genetic damage is known as *loss of heterozygosity*. It relates to aging and disease. But let's back up a second.

The DNA sequences of your 46 chromosomes contain more than 20,000 known coding genes (these are genes that carry the instructions for making proteins; they *code* for proteins) and a lot of other noncoding sequences that scientists don't yet understand. For any given gene except those located on the sex chromosomes in the case of men, you probably have two good copies of the same gene—that is, a maternal and a paternal *allele* (gene variant). An allele is one of the possible forms of a gene.

We call having two of the same alleles—one each from Mom and Dad—being *homozygous*. If there is a copy of a gene from one of your parents but not the other, we call that being *heterozygous* (having different alleles). For example, if you have the brown eye gene from Mom and the blue eye gene from Dad, you will have brown eyes because you are heterozygous and the brown eye gene variant, or allele, overpowers the blue one. That is known as a dominant versus recessive trait (though some traits, such as blood type, can show co-dominance). So, if you are heterozygous and mate with someone with blue eyes (who is by definition homozygous), your children will have a 50 percent chance of having blue eyes: the weaker trait of blue eyes needs two of the recessive alleles to be expressed.

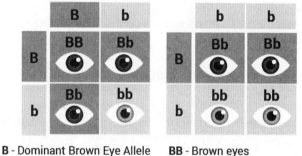

B - Dominant Brown Eye Allele   **BB** - Brown eyes
b - Recessive Blue Eye Allele   **Bb** - Brown eyes
                                      bb - Blue eyes

Some genetic "diseases" are relatively silent with heterozygosity, meaning that they probably won't manifest. Think of it as someone who has one healthy kidney instead of two; most people do fine with just one. For example, cystic fibrosis disease doesn't occur with one normal (aka "wild type") gene allele and one nonfunctioning one. Despite a 50 percent "gene dosage," cystic fibrosis is therefore called an *autosomal recessive* condition, meaning that the disease won't manifest unless you got zero wild type alleles. In other words, a parent can be an asymptomatic carrier of a cystic fibrosis gene and never know it unless he or she mates with another person who is also missing the normal cystic fibrosis gene. In that case, two carriers have offspring homozygous for non-functioning genes one out of four times.

On the other hand, some diseases present when there is only one good and one bad copy, referred to as an *autosomal dominant* disease condition, and that is bad news. We gave an example of this when we discussed one of the forms of premature aging, or *progeria*, known as *dyskeratosis congenita*. This disease results from having only one good copy of various components needed to operate telomerase.

What Is a Point Mutation?

We discussed that at a rate of about 0.32 times per cell division, we accumulate typographical errors in DNA that can then produce slightly different mRNAs and proteins or even render the transcripts untranslatable. When this happens, less-than-perfect or inadequate amounts of a crucial protein may be produced, resulting in misbehaving cells. Think changing one amino acid can't make a difference? Well, a single substitution of one amino acid can be the difference between normal blood hemoglobin and sickle cell anemia. However, if most of your genes are in order, these errors won't normally show up as disease, because sporadic mutants are outnumbered by your normal genes—unless, of course, you experience them in those immortal stem cells.

Here's another example of how genetic damage is acquired by aging. Let's say you lost the allele for the only good copy of a critical *oncogene* (a gene responsible for thwarting cells when they became damaged or don't play well with others). Then you might express a clinical cancer syndrome such as the infamous breast- and ovarian-cancer-associated conditions of BRCA1 and BRCA2.

An underappreciated notion among, patients, doctors, and even genetic experts is that even with two good copies of an allele, a stem cell can lose one functional allele and now express autosomal dominant disease conditions at the single cell level. If we only have one wild type allele, then loss of heterozygosity can confer full-blown expression of an autosomal recessive disease by taking us from aysmptomatic heterozygosity down to zero functioning copies of the critical allele. Given enough time, monkeys typing may not write Shakespeare, but chromosomes mutating will produce certain cell death every time. If you as an individual could survive every disease, you would eventually exhibit them all. Likewise, if your cells could survive every gene mutation, they would eventually acquire all possible mutations and disease states, because the genome can only get worse, not better, with copying and telomere-dysfunction induced mutations.

TELOMERE AND TELOMERASE
BASICS: THE LONG AND SHORT OF IT

Having mastered the basics of cell biology, genetics, and regular and stem cells, it's time to delve deeper into the heart of the matter: telomeres and telomerase.

As early as 1938, a geneticist named Hermann Muller first correctly intuited the role of the telomere:

> The terminal gene must have a special function, that
> of *sealing the end of the chromosome*, so to speak, and . . .
> for some reason a chromosome cannot persist indefinitely
> without having its ends thus sealed.[3] [emphasis added]

Muller correctly deduced that the terminal genes or ends of every chromosome, which he named the *telomeres* (remember: *telo*=end, *mere*=body), serve to protect the precious DNA libraries between them from being damaged. Without telomeres to protect DNA, chromosomes would be spliced into mutant double chromosomes by double-stranded DNA breakage repair, and this would beget chromosome confetti, or chromothripsis.

In 2009, the Nobel Prize committee awarded three scientists the honor in medicine and physiology for the discovery of telomerase, the enzyme used to relengthen telomeres. While this brought telomeres and their function into a new light, it wasn't the first time telomeres had been noted in the scientific community.

The existence of the end-replication problem was first formulated in Moscow by Alexey Olovnikov in 1971, 38 years before three scientists won a Nobel Prize for "discovering" telomerase. Olovnikov predicted a special compensatory DNA polymerase to counteract telomere shortening from cell replication in reproductive and cancer cells, whereas in most cells this would be inhibited, leading to cellular aging and the Hayflick limit.

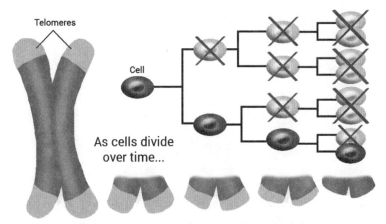

...telomeres shorten and eventually cell division stops

TELOMERASE REVERSES AGING

The big news in all of this is that the discovery of telomerase in immortal mama stem cells shows that the enzyme can actively lengthen and preserve telomeres, slowing or reversing aging at a cellular and symptomatic level. If your stem cells' telomeres are shortening, it shows that the telomerase system is failing to keep up with its task. Perhaps it is your stress, lack of exercise, or poor sleep that is hindering your stem cells from repairing?

Spoiler alert: that is the premise of this book.

While the telomerase gene is present in all cells, this micro-machine is only expressed in stem cells. Telomerase is made of a master protein—a nanomachine—called telomerase reverse transcriptase (TERT) that uses a ribonucleic acid (RNA) template add-on known as telomerase-associated RNA component (TERC) to rebuild and preserve telomeres. TERC and TERT cooperate to add back more DNA telomere length using an RNA template, six base pairs at a time. That's why it's referred to as *reverse* transcription because it is the *reverse* of the central dogma of DNA→RNA.

Telomerase, TERC and dyskerin all need to be present for telomere lengthening to occur

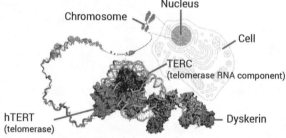

Telomerase itself can't be taken orally—it's a large protein and would be digested by the acid and protein destroyers in your digestive system. Telomerase can't be injected either—it's too big to diffuse into cells for use. So telomerase must be assembled for use only within the stem cell that uses it. *That's why the only effective way to activate telomerase is to do healthy things that enhance its functioning inside your body (or possibly ingest a molecule that elicits increased activity, as discussed in Chapter 9).*

Measuring Telomeres

Although most studies on telomeres assume that telomere lengths correspond to a person's age, it's far from that simple. This is like trying to estimate the age of a car based on the age of the oil filter—though the filter is changed much more frequently than the car. But in this analogy, there is a master oil filter that also ages very slowly, causing each replacement filter to start off with a little more wear and tear. That is why the general trend in all people for all organs appears to be one of shortening telomeres over their lifetimes. That said, there can be massive variation in telomere length between individuals of the same age and even within the same person in different organs or when measured at different times. The largest study of over 100,000 patients in the Kaiser system showed that in general, telomeres tend to shorten over time and that length variability increases as people grow older.

Measurable telomere shortening is a statistical artifact based on a dynamic situation, like measuring the water level in 46 bathtubs that are being slowly drained. In this analogy, non-stem cells can only drain some bathtubs; the mama queen stem cells are able to clone themselves with a full water level that actually gets refilled. Luckily, as with any good bathtub, there appears to be an overflow mechanism preventing the overlengthening of telomeres, as we can infer from people who have taken telomerase activators without adverse effects for more than nine years, and from certain trees that live happily for thousands of years with high telomerase activity.[4]

So, telomere length is a snapshot based upon which cells are being sampled; the more recent a cell's origination from the longer-telomere-having stem cell mama, the longer its telomeres will be. But over time, even the stem cell mama can develop shorter telomeres so the lifelong downward trend can be understood in that way.

THE TELOMERE MIRACLE IN A NUTSHELL

The answer to aging is simple—if we can figure out how to activate and amplify telomerase, we can reverse and stop aging. Now that you understand as much as, if not much more than, most doctors about genetics and cell biology, let's review my theory of aging.

My Telomere and Stem Cell Theory of Aging

- **Axiom 1:**
  Telomeres always shorten when one cell divides into two, and when telomeres become critically short, the cell malfunctions and/or dies from resulting chromosome mutation.

- **Axiom 2:**
  Non-stem cells cannot reproduce indefinitely.

- **Axiom 3:**
  A daughter cell can only be as healthy (genetic integrity) or as young (telomere length) as the stem cell it came from.

- **Axiom 4:**
  Stem cells can restore telomere length with telomerase.

- **Hypothesis:**
  Aging is caused by the shortening of telomeres in stem cells. Therefore, if telomerase activity increases in stem cells, then telomere length will be preserved and the effects of aging will be slowed and possibly reversed.

In the next chapter, we'll discuss how the current science misinterprets aging, we'll delve deeper into the real reason you get old, and we'll discuss the one cure for aging as we know it.

Chapter 3

Aging—One Cause, One Cure

Intuition is the royal road to wisdom.

Ask people to describe aging and they might tell you about what doctors call *symptoms* (aka patients' subjective complaints): sagging and dry skin, thinning and gray hair, inability to read up close, weight gain, achy and stiff joints, loss of desire and sexual performance, and fogginess and forgetfulness.

Or, you might present with what physicians refer to as *signs* (aka things identified, or prompted from the patient, by the doctor): wrinkles, pattern baldness, stiff eye lenses, belly fat, limited limb range due to tenderness and stiffness, slowed reflexes, vaginal dryness or erectile dysfunction, and poor concentration and memory recall.

Or, a doctor might give you a list of *conditions, diagnoses,* or *diseases* that you've been labeled with: photoaging (sun-damaged skin), alopecia (hair loss), presbyopia (farsightedness), obesity, degenerative joint disease, menopause or "andropause" (for the hombres), and Alzheimer's disease.

But what if I told you that whatever it's called—whether a subjective complaint, an observable sign, or a full-blown disease diagnosis—it's all related to the same thing?

SO, WHAT'S THE REAL REASON WE GET OLD?

Today, almost all humans experience similar problems as they get chronologically older, because all people are made up of cells that contain the same genetic machinery and operated by the same ground rules that we described in the previous chapter. Here, I invoke Occam's razor, a problem-solving principle attributed to 14th-century English monk and philosopher William of Ockham, which states that when one simple explanation will suffice, don't evoke multiple complex ones. In other words, when you hear hoofbeats, think horses, not zebras chasing unicorns. Keep it simple.

In fact, if you go to your doctor for a checkup, especially if you are north of 40, chances are that many of your complaints—weight gain, a shortage of energy, aches and pains in various body parts, high blood pressure and cholesterol, difficulty sleeping, and so on—will usually be normalized by your friendly family physician, if not dismissed outright, as part of the aging process. Your doctor might note your signs and symptoms as separate problems, yet throw them all under the category of ordinary aging. Your doctor will likely explain to you that it's all part of one inevitable process—aging—but won't grasp that these signs, symptoms, and diseases can be united under one simple theory (as previously mentioned).

In all probability you will leave your appointment with a prescription and/or suggestions to exercise, stretch, supplement with hormones, lower your dietary fat and sodium levels, or take other medications to control blood pressure and cholesterol. But any consideration of addressing a common cause (the shortening of telomeres) and a single remedy (the preservation of telomeres) for these shared, coincident, and progressive signs, symptoms, and diseases is something you'll never hear from your doctor.

How Do Scientists Misinterpret Aging?

If asked, most scientists who study aging and clinicians who practice the various subspecialties related to aging would tell you they haven't ever actually considered that there could be one overarching explanation for the many afflictions of growing old. It's like going to a mechanic who tells you he or she has never once considered that the rust in your car's brakes could be the same as the rust that erodes the cylinders of the same machine. It's like an astrophysicist telling you he or she has never considered that the same principle that makes Venus rotate around the sun is similar to the one that makes Earth also rotate around the sun. Apparently, there are no points awarded for simplicity or originality when it comes to opinions about aging.

Instead, experts believe that each sign, symptom, condition, or disease associated with aging must have a unique cause that requires its own chemical pathway—one that can be mitigated by some billion-dollar, FDA-approved wonder drug. Some experts will even propose, with a straight face, that balding and growing a fat gut evolved because these were perceived as high-status cues to potential mates.

Part of the fault comes from the reductive and rote nature of medical education. To be competent, a physician doesn't learn about "joint trauma" but rather the unique types of injuries to ankles, shoulders, and other tendons and joints. Doctors and scientists are required to master specific diagnoses and treatments, not to understand proper body alignment and injury prevention in general. In other words, most medical professionals (and most of us) don't look at the big picture—how your cells hold the key to avoiding all these signs, symptoms, and diseases of aging!

The strange bias toward believing in infinite diseases and the promise of undiscovered magic bullets permeates all our notions of aging and is the reason no one questions the "many reasons for rust" mode of thinking. My Telomere Stem Cell Theory of Aging is so simple and obvious that most people will (wrongly) conclude that it couldn't possibly be true, because no one else is saying it.

Therefore, the absence of anyone quoting my adage "There is only one disease with many faces" implies that I am mistaken, not just ahead of my time. It is much like the absence of a dialogue about a heliocentric solar system, which was rendered as fringe thinking for most of our recorded scientific and philosophical history.

Some researchers believe, despite the lack of verifiable research, that there must be signaling pathways such as sirtuins (a class of regulatory proteins) stimulated by the antioxidant resveratrol to combat aging (the popular drink-red-wine-fountain-of-youth theory). After much expense and much research, the idea of activating the sirtuin gene to improve health and longevity has been abandoned, because of safety concerns and lack of efficacy across all indications of use, by the same pharmaceutical company that previously paid $720 million to purchase this business. In just one of many studies, Johns Hopkins researchers recently followed 783 older men and women in Tuscany for nine years, measuring their wine intake by urinanalysis. Then they divided the population into quartiles based on amounts of resveratrol metabolites. The percentage of people who died was exactly the same from highest to lowest intakes of resveratrol.[1]

Other anti-aging gurus propose that free radicals and oxidative damage from mitochondria cause aging and that the taking of antioxidants is the cure. Not so fast. In a McGill University study, researchers reported that even when antioxidants naturally produced inside of cells are disabled (they did this to worms), the antioxidant-depleted subjects unexpectedly lived 30 percent longer than those with active antioxidants.[2] Other studies show that supplementing with antioxidants, as we will discuss in Chapter 9, doesn't postpone aging.[3] The takeaway here is that supplementing with antioxidants probably doesn't help, and may potentially harm, your health.

So what is the answer to aging? So what does every "new sheriff in town" share? A business plan, credibility, investors, and products to sell. Instead of trying something new, I propose that we use what we already have within our bodies—telomerase—activated by the natural youth-preserving TeloMirror Tools that you'll learn to incorporate into your life in Part II. But first, let's go back to the real reason you get old.

THERE IS ONLY ONE DISEASE WITH A THOUSAND FACES

Despite its many facets, all we think of as being associated with growing old and most of the diseases that accompany it, can be explained by one root cause:

Aging is the result of DNA damage caused by the telomere shortening that occurs in stem cells over time.

Ah, we return to my hypothesis. Yes. I believe that all forms of disease and symptoms of aging can be accounted for by the malfunction and destruction of DNA caused by the critical shortening of telomeres. In study after study, shorter telomeres have been associated with heart disease, Alzheimer's, arthritis, osteoporosis, macular degeneration, liver failure, skin damage, and AIDS. You name the complaint or disease and it's likely that it can be traced back to cellular and organ dysfunction caused by loss of telomere length.

It is critical that you know that all premature-aging diseases found in nature involve errors in DNA integrity or cell replication. This strongly suggests that the fundamental drivers of aging and disease are problems of data-integrity preservation.

There are no models of premature aging that would support the multibillion-dollar "moonshots" led by venture capitalists and celebrity scientists. Sadly, the cure for aging is not being approached like an engineering problem. If I wanted to build a flying machine, it might behoove me to study how nature has solved the engineering problem in multiple species, learn aerodynamics and how to machine engineering, and then do some thinking, planning, and experimenting around natural systems. We are made, maintained, and repaired using stem cells, and those cells copy a lot and require efficient and faithful DNA replication and telomere maintenance.

Why not consider a telomere/stem cell cause for aging and disease? Follow the money. Academics, think-tankers, venture capitalists, and entrepreneurs can't monetize a universal cause and cure for aging that we already possess in every stem cell, so the telomere theory of aging doesn't get the attention it deserves.

> *It is difficult to get a man to understand something,*
> *when his salary depends upon his not understanding it!*
> *— Upton Sinclair*

THE SINGLE SOLUTION TO AGING

Speaking of the medical-academic-industrial complex, here are just a few of the thousands of studies suggesting the ubiquitous influence of telomeres on aging and various symptoms, signs, and diseases associated with aging:

- The *Heart* of the Matter: High levels of **stress,** elevated stress hormones, **smoking, high blood pressure,** high blood sugar, **prediabetic markers,** high levels of **belly fat,** and **heart disease** risk were all linked to low telomerase activity among 62 women, ages 35 to 41, in a study published in the journal *Psychoneuroendocrinology.* The University of California–San Francisco researchers did urine and blood tests to determine the health markers and telomerase levels and also had the women report their levels of mental stress. Based on all the health issues noted, the researchers conclude that low telomerase is an early marker of heart-disease risk.[4]

- A *Weighty* Issue: London investigators recruited more than 1,100 women, ages 18 to 76, measured their telomeres, and recorded their weight status. They found that lean women had longer telomeres, while **overweight** and **obese** women had much shorter ones. Obtaining or maintaining a healthy weight preserves the health of your telomeres, concluded the researchers from the University of Medicine and Dentistry and St. Thomas Hospital in London.[5]

- A *Joint* Perspective: Average telomere length is not only shorter in those with **arthritis**, it's ultra-short where the damage is most severe, according to Danish researchers. In a small but highly accurate study published in *Arthritis Research and Therapy,* investigators tested the telomere length in DNA cartilage of 14 osteoarthritis patients who were having knee-replacement surgery. Not only was the average telomere length shorter when compared to nine adults of the same age without arthritis, telomere length appeared progressively shorter in the cells that were closer to the arthritic area.[6]

- A *Dense* Subject: King's College London researchers found that of 2,150 women, ages 18 to 79, those who were at risk for **osteoporosis** and had poorer **bone density** had shorter telomeres than women who were at low risk for the condition. In the study, published in *Osteoporosis International*, the researchers found the link between telomere length and weakened bone by measuring samples from the spines and forearms of the women. They concluded that telomere length is a likely marker of bone aging.[7]

- An *Age-Defying* Act: When Harvard researchers genetically engineered mice that lacked the ability to produce telomerase, they saw accelerated symptoms of aging, including organ failure, tissue injury, gray hair, and wrinkled skin. The study, published in *Nature,* was the first to then show the reversing effects of telomerase: The researchers injected the no-telomerase mice to reactivate the enzyme, and they saw these same effects of aging reverse. Gray hair became dark, wrinkled skin smoothed and plumped, energy returned, and organs regained function.[8] In another longevity study, published in the *Proceedings of the National Academy of Sciences*, researchers found that centenarians (people living to be 100 or older) had unusually high telomerase activity compared to those who died at younger ages.[9]

IF OUR STEM CELLS ALREADY HAVE TELOMERASE, WHY DO WE AGE AT ALL?

In Hindu mythology, there are three deities referred to as the *trimurti* (or three forms). First, there is the creator god, Brahma. Second, there is the sustainer, Vishnu. Finally, there is the god of destruction, Shiva. Let us borrow from this model to interpret how aging and illness arises from the interplay between all three processes of creation, maintenance, and destruction.

Birth: Consider our master stem cells as like the deity of Brahma, the creator. We mentioned my "Redenbacher effect" of getting many different diseases in our advanced age as the result of a shared common stem cell ancestry from available mesenchymal stem cell reserves that have been depleted in number and degraded in quality over the course of a lifetime of replicative senescence and potential mutagens. If you sample bone marrow from an old person, you'll find fewer stem cells and less diversity as well as less integrity with respect to the original genomic code. Throughout life, we become less like ourselves, because local and source stem cells acquire errors; we become genetically mosaic, so that instead of one version of DNA, we have many versions with many more epigenetic programs that act like malware.

Maintenance: Let's talk about Vishnu, the preserver, represented by telomerase and its attempted maintenance of existing stem cells. In times of high replicative burden, we can't always keep up with the escalator, and we experience shortening of telomeres without compensatory relengthening. Even with perfect telomere maintenance, the low level of typographical errors as well as other forms of genetic and epigenetic changes can lead to a situation where we don't actually want those bad stem cells to keep surviving. Part of the reason our cells and we grow old is that unlike other mammals, we can. Our cells and bodies are able to function despite suboptimal cellular programing and integrity.

Destruction: Finally, there is the creative destruction of Lord Shiva. Luckily, every cell has many mechanisms to recognize genetic damage, and this either halts replication or provokes cell suicide, known as apoptosis. Studies of compounds that inhibit the inhibitors of stem cell suicide show that enhancing cell death not only cures cancer (damaged stem cells) but also reverses aging in animal models. This rapid destruction of damaged cells is a potential double-edged sword, however, because we don't know if it will accelerate depletion of our reserves of relatively pristine stem cells.

A Bathtub Analogy and the *Trimurti* Reinterpreted

Think of your body and your life as a pleasant bathing experience, with the water representing cells. When you are young, the water enters the tub cleanly. Over time, the recycled water becomes soiled, so it can be filtered or drained. Despite constant waste being excreted into the bathtub by you, we hope to maintain a comfortable and sanitary experience, even though you're bathing in a tub filled with water/cells that have varying levels of health, dysfunction, and outright disease.

The creative principle of Brahma is like the fresh water, in the form of stem cells. We humans have a stem cell ecology that prevents us from having excessively high proportions of stem cells, unlike some immortal invertebrates with high percentages of stem cells, like the giant squid or jellyfish, which can grow huge forever because they don't need to keep stable in the wind (like trees) or worry about size overgrowth (like humans in studio apartments and old jeans and shoes). To keep from overflowing the tub, our bodies have a spillover valve; that is the internal set point for the number of stem cell niches that can coexist in our post-pubertal, one-size-for-life bodies/bathtubs.

Now we have the principle of Vishnu, the preserver. If we have nearly 100 percent telomerase activity, it is likely that slightly dysfunctional versions of our local stem cells accumulate, leading to the senescent cells and their behaviors that manifest as disease and aging. On the one hand, preservation of stem cells slows the cataclysmic mutation caused by end-to-end fusions, but on the other hand, point mutations, loss of homo- and heterozygosity, and epigenetic malware will invariably ensue. If the same water is maintained too long, it becomes polluted, but that's better than having an empty tub.

Finally, we have the senolytic, apoptic, and destructive ability to remove debris (like using a goldfish net to remove poop during a home birth) and the ability to open the drain up and flush out the polluted water. The destruction of Lord Shiva, represented by cell death and cell removal, is a good thing, but only if we also somewhat maintain the water level and introduce fresh water. Exercise and intermittent fasting produce healthy, low-level destruction, whereas cancer chemotherapy and infections represent accelerated destruction.

In order to enjoy an eternal bath in relatively clean bathing conditions, we need a fresh supply of water. Unfortunately, our bone marrow MSCs deplete and we can't yet freeze and thaw them reliably. We also need good water-level maintenance, and luckily our two copies of telomerase systems running in each cell keep us filled up for 80-something years. Finally, we need to actively filter the water and drain it by mastering apoptosis and autophagy without pulling the plug for too long, as occurs with chronic viral infections that deplete our immune systems or cancer chemotherapy that drains the water too quickly by massive stem cell extinction events.

My simple idea is that the damage to stem cells, largely caused by telomere attrition and mutation, is the root of aging and disease. I believe this will someday seem as obvious as the notion that we are revolving around the sun, despite it being clear for all to see in the sky that the opposite might be true.

WHAT'S NEXT?

We've covered a lot of information in these first three chapters. Let's pause for a moment and review the key points to remember:

- **The tools in this book are called TeloMirror Tools** because the benefits of your lifestyle choices are shown by science to be reflected by the health of your telomeres.

- **Because of the mechanics of DNA replication**, telomeres always grow shorter when cells divide.

- **Ordinary, non-stem cells must die.** This is called the Hayflick limit, and it serves to protect us from expendable rogue cell lines that have become mutated or defective.

- **Stem cells are capable of regrowing shortened telomeres** with telomerase, and in perfect conditions, they can live forever, although we want damaged ones to die as well. When damaged stem cells don't die off, we get dysfunctional cells and are prone to cancer and disease.

- **Telomeres are dynamic.** They can lengthen or shorten in stem cells as a function of telomerase activation, overcopying, and environmental effects (aka how you live your life).

- **Ordinary cells cannot be younger or healthier** than their most recent stem cell parent.

- **The health of your stem cells** equals the health of your cells and organs.

- **The shortening of telomeres in stem cells** causes aging, but it can be mitigated if telomeres in stem cells have adequate telomerase activation.

In the next six chapters, we will examine the TeloMirror Tools (TMTs) that play an essential role in slowing down the shortening of your telomeres by as yet unclear means. These tools are breathing, mind-set, sleep, exercise, diet, and supplements. At the risk of disappointing you, I will forewarn you that much of this content may seem obvious to some, but I'll bet that there will still be plenty of new facts, ideas, and even many "life hacks" that will fascinate you.

THE BIG PICTURE: THANK YOUR
PARENTS FOR THE LIFE SPAN YOU DO ENJOY

There's a simple reason we don't all die of old age when we're 14, like people with only a 50 percent gene dosage of the wild type telomerase allele encountered in certain autosomal dominant forms of dyskeratosis congenita (doesn't it feel good to understand that fancy sentence, by the way?).

Happily, your body's stem cells and their homozygous wild type gene dosage of telomerase activity are pretty good at keeping you young. Our goal in the following chapters will be to use the things you are already expert at, such as breathing, sleeping, thinking, and eating, in order to maximize the efficiency of that full gene dosage of telomerase and delay the stem cell depletion caused by the Redenbacher effect and the natural loss of numbers and quality of stem cells that we carry around.

The bad news? Unlike this chapter, which was mostly science orthodoxy with a smattering of theory, the following chapters may try your patience. Perhaps you might review my Author's Note: this ride has the potential to be a bit bumpy for those used to learning in an accretive fashion (adding to what they already know).

The following TeloMirror Toolbox chapters will require patience, a modicum of fresh thinking, and some faith in your intuition—the royal road to wisdom that has served Mendel, Olovnikov, and me so well.

PART II

TELOMIRRORS— THE TOOLS THAT TURN BACK TIME

It's time to get into the heart of our *TeloMirror Tools (TMTs)*. These individual tools—breathing, mind-set, sleep, exercise, diet, and supplements—work in harmony like the cylinders in a car engine. The purpose of a cylinder and its piston is to transfer force from that chamber's gasoline explosion to push the movable piston within it and help to drive something called the crankshaft. One piston can transfer only so much force, but six pistons all pushing the crankshaft can really create some horsepower. That's why a V8 engine (with eight cylinders in a V shape) creates more force than a four- or six-cylinder engine and a V12 is even stronger. To belabor the analogy, each piston can be optimized with fuel injection, precise timing, polishing off rust, and making sure the seals are good.

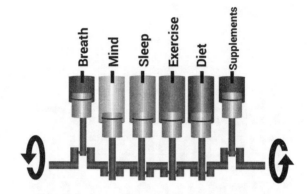

The next six chapters focus on each of the TMTs in turn and are structured similarly:

- The basic mechanics for the tool in question
- The purpose of each tool
- Common challenges and issues
- The available telomere science
- Best practices to leverage the power of each TMT

Ready? Let's get your anti-aging engine revved.

Chapter 4

Your Breath

Breathe in, breathe out. Repeat until death.

Breathing is the most crucial yet least considered aspect of living. Let me prove it.

Try this: stop and hold your breath for as long as you can right now.

Keep holding.

Keep holding.

How'd you do? Twenty seconds? A minute?

That's about how long most people can go without this particular tool.

WHY IS BREATHING THE TOP TMT?

You can survive weeks without eating and days without drinking and sleeping; but you will be alive for only minutes without the ability to breathe. No oxygen and excess carbon dioxide is lethal. Breathing is something that you do more than 20,000 times a day but rarely think about. What if we could learn to optimize breathing in each moment, each activity, and throughout a life? Surely this would only benefit our health and longevity.

We will gain insight into the system by asking a simple question: Why is it impossible to kill yourself by holding your breath?

1. You inhale oxygen into your lungs, and your lungs pass the oxygen into your bloodstream.

2. Your red blood cells carry the oxygen to your cells.

3. Your cells use oxygen from your blood to break down and transform glucose (that's what food is converted into after it is digested) into the energy your body needs to run its chemical machinery. This cellular respiration produces carbon dioxide and is always on.

4. When you exhale, you rid your blood of carbon dioxide that has accumulated.

5. If you hold your breath, you cut off oxygen and build up carbon dioxide, acidifying your blood.

6. The urge to breathe is so overpowering that I doubt there are any people who could voluntarily hold their breath even long enough to lose consciousness, let alone kill themselves. The job of breathing is too important to be entrusted to you. With or without you, low-oxygen and high-acidity sensors will resume breathing by signaling your primitive brainstem, the control room for your body.

BREATH IS LIFE

In the book of Genesis, the transfer of breath was literally the genesis of life, the *sine qua non* of being alive.

> *Then the LORD God formed the man out of the dust*
> *from the ground and breathed the breath of life into*
> *his nostrils, and the man became a living being.*
> *— Genesis 2:7*

In the ancient proto-Hindi language of Sanskrit, one word for breath is *prana*, which can also be loosely translated as "life force." My point here is that people grasped the central role of breathing long before respiratory science, neuroscience, and brain imaging.

Sadly, despite all the science and wisdom surrounding breathing, most of us shortchange ourselves with just about every breath we take, and when you don't breathe properly, you are probably aging faster. It doesn't have to be this way. As you'll learn, by implementing simple breathing techniques, you can slow aging and increase both the quantity and quality of your life.

On the following pages, you'll learn a little about getting the most out of the 12 to 20 breaths you take each and every minute of your life. First, we'll look at just what breathing is, more about the purpose and worth of breathing, the mechanics of how your body breathes, and what telomere science says about breathing. Then we'll explore the most common problems people have with breathing. We'll talk about some simple fixes and finally wrap up with the best ways to incorporate healthier breathing into your life.

WHAT IS THE PURPOSE OF BREATHING?

As I alluded to, there are two main reasons for breathing: to take in oxygen and to expel carbon dioxide. Let's take a moment to understand why.

Oxygen

In a confusing bit of shared terminology, our body's respiration serves to support *cellular respiration*. Cellular respiration is the process by which your cells transform blood sugar, aka glucose, into something called *adenosine triphosphate* (ATP). You may vaguely recall from high school biology that oxidative phosphorylation occurs in the mitochondria of our cells, and perhaps you've retained some crucial terms like *glycolysis* and the *Krebs cycle*.

Don't worry, we won't make you relearn this. Oxygen is required to make ATP, and ATP is the universal fuel for living systems.

In a sense, cellular respiration works like the change machine you'd find in a Laundromat. In this analogy, the washing machines only operate on quarters. Here, you can think of ATP as the quarters that all the machines in our bodies run on. By eating, we acquire the large bills of sugars, proteins, and dietary fat, but these currencies are useless for doing laundry because the machines need quarters (ATP). All the dietary fat, protein, and sugars that you ever eat, make, or store must first be converted to dollars (glucose), which is then fed into the change machine (cellular respiration) to get those ATP quarters.

Our cellular "machines" only run on the "coins" of ATP

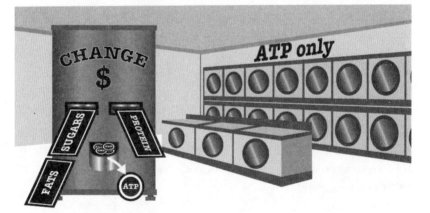

Carbon Dioxide

The other purpose of your breathing is to get rid of the waste by-product of cellular respiration, which is carbon dioxide (CO_2); in a sense, you exhale because your cells need to exhale. If you don't exhale adequately to blow off the CO_2, it quickly builds up as carbonic acid in your body and makes your system too acidic. Your entire biochemistry—your cells and your organs—cannot operate properly if your system is too acidic.

Breathing Regulates Your pH

You may have heard the term *pH level* (pH=potential of hydrogen) because we use it to describe things like swimming pools, blood, and cleaning solutions. The pH scale is a logarithmic scale from 1 to 14 that quantifies the balance between acidity and alkalinity in any solution. A neutral pH is 7, and every number lower than 7 indicates a solution is 10 times more acidic, whereas every number greater than 7 indicates 10 times less acidic (aka more basic/alkaline).

It is imperative that we maintain our blood system's pH within a narrow and slightly alkaline range—7.35 to 7.45. We are beings that require balance, and this goes for pH levels too. By definition, the lower your pH, the higher your acidity and presence of hydrogen atoms. The higher your pH, the fewer free hydrogen atoms you have and the more alkaline your blood becomes. Being outside of this narrow range is incompatible with life, which is a big reason we breathe.

Achieving pH balance through diet and alkaline water is a popular but oversimplified notion. While nutrition, fluid intake, and your kidneys do help determine your body's pH level, the most important way you regulate your pH in real time is by exhaling CO_2 and monitoring pH via sensors connected to the brain stem (which controls breathing). Something as simple as running for a short burst can build up acid from cellular metabolism of ATP and glucose. A few deep breaths release the acidity-spiking CO_2 and quickly put you back into the safe zone.

On the flip side, your pH can swing the other way and become too basic if you hyperventilate (breathe too rapidly). Rapid breathing blows off too much CO_2, which causes blood pH to rise above 7.45 and results in dizziness, tingling, muscle spasms, and other distressing symptoms. Don't worry, though; it is very difficult to get into trouble through hyperventilation—with the notable and illustrative exception of something called "shallow-water drowning." Swimmers who are training to hold their breath for longer times intentionally breathe rapidly to blow off CO_2 and raise their blood pH. Because of this buffer of higher pH, the buildup of CO_2 and acidification of the blood is delayed and the critical signal to breathe isn't triggered. This can cause the swimmer to lose consciousness. Eventually oxygen gets so low that the low-oxygen sensors do trigger the unconscious body to inhale water, and drowning happens.

Of course, shallow-water drowning and trying to hold your breath until you die are unusual circumstances. In the course of our real lives, breathing is safe and automatic. But that doesn't mean you can't optimize your health by focusing on mindful, relaxing, focused, and balanced breathing. A recurring theme with this and all the TMTs is that, when it comes to the human body, balance preserves telomeres and helps to create healthier, longer lives.

HOW DOES BREATHING WORK?

Just remember what you've been taught about breathing!

Of course, I'm just kidding. While the popularity of meditation and yoga has grown—and both usually include some directions for how to breathe—I'm fairly certain that you never had formal instruction in how to breathe. The majority of breathing that you do is done automatically and unconsciously. But learning the strategies of the TMT of breathing will not only improve your exchange of gases and regulation of pH, it may help preserve your telomeres and increase telomerase activity by keeping your cells happy and in balance, possibly by activating the endocannabinoid system.

Science is just beginning to understand the wide-ranging effects of this group of cannabinoid receptors found in the brain. As you probably know, this system can be externally activated by two active molecules found in marijuana: THC (tetrahydrocannabinol) and CBD (cannabidiol). However, there's an internal activation system as well. Your body makes two marijuana-similar chemicals, original and natural neurotransmitters that are active when we feel "high on life." We intrinsically make anandamide (from the Sanskrit word for "joy" or "bliss") that binds the CBD1 receptor as THC does. We also intrinsically make 2-arachidonoyl-glycerol (2-AG) that binds to both CBD1 and CBD2 receptors like its marijuana-derived analogue, CBD.

Plant-derived cannabinoids

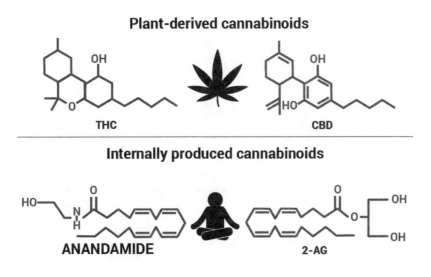

THC

CBD

Internally produced cannabinoids

ANANDAMIDE

2-AG

What does this have to do with the breathing TMT? Effective, and especially mindful, breathing activates the endocannabinoid system. (I'll come back to this in Chapter 9 to discuss herbal extracts that can enhance endocannabinoid signaling.) But in truth, all benefits of TeloMirror practices are potentially acting via the endocannabinoid system. Deep breathing, meditation, deep sleep, runner's high, eating chocolate cake—they all keep you young, because when you're experiencing all those "good vibrations," your cells are also feeling the love via endocannabinoid signaling.

Let's briefly recap: Oxygen (O_2) goes to your lungs and then into your blood, where it is carried throughout the body. Your cells and their mitochondria use oxygen to transform food energy into the tokens (ATP) that your cells need to function. Then you exhale the waste product of carbon dioxide (CO_2). That's the big picture, but now what are the mechanics?

THE MECHANICS AND MUSCLE OF BREATHING

Inhaling and exhaling: There are three ways to inhale, presented here in order of decreasing efficiency. Most efficient is having the dome-shaped muscular sheet at the bottom of your chest, called the diaphragm, drop down, creating a vacuum and sucking in air. Next, you can use the muscles between the ribs to lift and expand the rib cage, again creating a vacuum. Finally, to breathe in extra hard, there are muscles known as accessory muscles of respiration in your neck and shoulders that can lift the rib cage a bit more to suck in even more air by expanding, like an accordionist really stretching his arms out for a long note. When we are sleeping or exercising, we breathe efficiently. In contrast, when we are self-consciously inhaling, we tend to use our chest and rib breathing, and when we are anxious, we only take little sips with our accessory muscles, resulting in shoulder and neck pain.

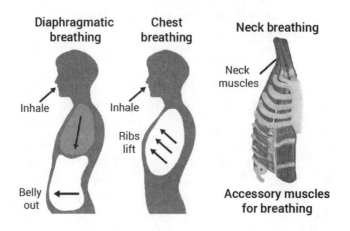

Breathing out is usually the result of passive recoil of your elastic rib cage after being stretched outward (the way a rubber band retracts after being stretched). But the diaphragm, abdominal muscles, and the muscles between ribs can also actively help to expel the air more efficiently if or when that is called for.

Breathing is fascinating because it is under three different levels of control—automatic, semivoluntary, and voluntary control.

First, there's the automatic drive to breathe, which you can't stop unless you damage your brain stem, overdose on opioids, or experience carbon monoxide poisoning. Even people in comas who have massive brain damage to the reasoning centers of the cerebral cortex will continue breathing automatically because of signals that come from the more "primitive" brain stem.

Normally, there is no "off switch" for breathing, just as your heart also beats automatically, involuntarily, and continuously. There is an improvised "off switch" used in certain situations: the *coup de grâce*, or "graceful blow," that refers to a form of mercy killing. The term comes from chivalric battle. In medieval battle, a knight's armor was so heavy that if he fell from his horse, he couldn't easily even get up, so he was probably going to be easily vanquished. In bullfighting, an animal that is mortally wounded and simply bleeding to death is no longer entertaining, I suppose. In both instances, a coup de grâce severing the brain stem at the base of the skull serves to halt the involuntary control of breathing and heart rate.

Next, we have semivoluntary control of our breathing. Let's say that you are hiding in a closet from a serial killer. Even though your panic system wants you to breathe rapidly to fuel your escape, you may have the ability to override this automatic system and breathe quietly. If you feel disappointed or frustrated, you might decide to sigh deeply and audibly, both to subconsciously relax and perhaps to express your feelings to those nearby to hear it. In both these cases, your breathing is at least partially under your control, not completely automatic, and not completely conscious and voluntary—so it is semivoluntary.

Voluntary breathing is done intentionally by turning your mental focus upon your breath. I would venture a guess that 99.9999 percent of all your breathing is done without conscious thought. But mindful breathing can change your physical and mental state in much the same way body language can. Stand up straight or put on a big smile and you can transform your internal state (how you feel) as well as how people perceive you (how they feel about you). By consciously focusing on your breathing, you can instantly improve your mindfulness, mood, balance, and sense of well-being. There is a reason that many meditation techniques focus on breathing: if you keep your focus on your breath, you'll be much more likely to stay in the present, dynamic moment, not the stories of the past or the imagined future.

WHAT DOES TELOMERE SCIENCE TELL US ABOUT BREATHING?

As discussed in Chapter 1, when looking at just about any age-related decline in health or formation of disease, researchers nearly always uncover a connection to shorter telomeres, lower telomerase activity, or both. This will be a theme repeated as we move through all the TMTs, and it is certainly true of telomeres and your respiratory system. Scientists who study telomeres and lung function have found a relationship between better breathing and longer telomeres. Similarly, researchers have found a link between diseases of the respiratory system and shorter telomeres and lower telomerase activity.

- **Chronic lung disease shows mutated telomerase.** In a Johns Hopkins University study, researchers found that when people have telomerase gene mutations (remember, we already discussed that this causes prematurely shortened telomeres; see page 40), they rapidly developed a crippling lung condition known as idiopathic pulmonary fibrosis (IPF). People with IPF have lungs that are thick, stiff, and scarred. The researchers recruited more than 600 people, each with one family member who was identified as having IPF. Not only did the IPF people have telomerase mutated genes and shorter telomeres, than compared to people who were disease free, the IPF sufferers were more likely to have family members who inherited this telomerase gene mutation. Based on these findings, the family members with the mutations are at risk for shorter telomeres and IPF.[1]

Comment: Even with a full gene dosage of telomerase, all our lungs deteriorate starting in young adulthood. Breath is life and accelerated loss of breath means accelerated loss of life (i.e., aging). It is compelling that telomerase gene mutations are directly and causally related to both global premature aging and lung aging or fibrosis. Perhaps better breathing and telomerase activity can slow aging generally and declining respiratory function specifically?

- **Smoking causes increase in telomere shortening.** It has been established in scientific papers that mutations in telomerase and telomere genes cause abnormal telomere shortening. In a study from Johns Hopkins University, researchers found such mutations in smokers with severe emphysema.[2]

  Comment: The direct toxic effects from smoking might cause chromosomal mutation of stem cells (recall the loss of heterozygosity from Chapter 2). But there is possibly even greater mutation in stem cells from the higher-than-normal replicative senescence required to address the higher turnover from inflammation and tissue destruction caused by smoking. Just like an alcoholic's liver ages faster from overuse than a teetotaler's, a smoker's lungs age and become damaged from more rapid stem cell copying without adequate telomere restoration time.

- **Chronic lung disease severely increases telomere shortening.** *Chronic obstructive pulmonary disease* (COPD) is an umbrella term used to describe progressive lung diseases including emphysema, chronic bronchitis, refractory (nonreversible) asthma, and some forms of bronchiectasis. According to Danish researchers who tested the telomere lengths in more than 46,000 adults, shorter telomere lengths are 28 times more common in those with COPD than in those who don't have this lung disease.[3]

Comment: Once again, there's no denying that shorter telomere lengths are strongly associated with lung disease.

- **COPD damages telomeres and telomerase activity.** In a review and comparison of 14 studies, German researchers found that both COPD and asthma were correlated with shorter telomere length. The authors concluded that "cellular senescence may contribute to the pathogenesis of COPD and asthma, and that lung function may reflect biological aging primarily due to intrinsic processes, which are likely to be aggravated in lung diseases."[4]

  Comment: In other words, the diseases of aging (in this case COPD and asthma) are really caused by the same thing—telomere shortening.

- **Lung disease reversed with telomerase activator.** Now for a bit of good news from a study by researchers at the University of Texas Health Science Center, the University of Hawaii, the John A. Burns School of Medicine, and scientists from Geron Corporation. The investigators were able to reverse the effects of IPF (the "incurable" lung condition mentioned in the first study) when they introduced a telomerase activator to mice with the condition.[5]

  Comment: This important experiment takes a well-described incurable syndrome and specifically ameliorates the genetic shortcoming with a chemical inducer of telomerase. These are the kinds of studies validating the clinical use of telomerase activators, which we will discuss in Chapter 9.

It appears that science is backing up the ancients' claims that breath is life. At birth your lungs are not fully mature; it takes time for them to develop. Your lungs reach maximum efficiency in your 20s and then gradually decline. With each passing year, our lungs move less air, less efficiently, and with poorer diffusion. This downward trend is the same in measurable arterial function, skin elasticity, hair and nail growth, and sexual function. If we're being honest, the only thing that objectively improves after your 20s is your opinion of yourself.

So, studies show that lung disease is associated with shorter telomeres, but what if diminished breathing is both a result and a cause of aging? A result, because the lungs are made of cells (including niche stem lung cells) that also undergo accumulated telomere stem cell damage with inadequate repair and replacement; a cause, because we are breathing on behalf of all our cells, and over time, your cells suffer the adverse effects of inefficient oxygen and CO_2 exchange. Since most studies don't look at lung-specific telomeres, but instead at the easy-to-measure telomeres in blood cells, this general cause of aging from poor respiratory function is well supported.

Although certain conditions can accelerate telomere erosion in the lungs, such as exposure to toxins like smoke and air pollution, it is probably the deterioration of stem cell genomic integrity local to the lung and generally in the reserve bone marrow that causes us to lose functional lung capacity year after year. The lungs are made up of air tubes and sacs, spongy tissue, blood vessels, and an immune system. But efficient breathing also requires good biomechanics, which are a function of bones, muscles, joints, and ligaments. What do all these tissues have in common? They all come from stem cells that undergo telomere attrition and are subject to chromosomal mutation.

IS THERE A WRONG WAY TO BREATHE?

I started off this chapter by suggesting that most of us shortchange ourselves in the breathing department and that incorrect breathing ages you faster. Learning how to breathe to stay younger begins by becoming aware of the ways in which you may be breathing yourself older. It seems absurd to think we need to learn how to breathe, but is it really?

Why Do Many People Breathe Wrong When Told to "Take a Deep Breath"?

If I were to start recording you with a video camera and asked you to take a deep breath, you'd most likely expand your chest and suck UP your diaphragm, causing your belly to suck in. I learned this as a doctor, asking countless patients to take a deep breath during exams. Perhaps, to the mind's eye, that's what a deep breath is supposed to look like, but it really is just a bad actor's version of breathing.

When you move air correctly, as you would while swimming, singing, or sleeping restfully, you breathe into your abdomen first, which must expand down, causing your belly to protrude rather than retract. A healthy breath of air is similar to water flowing into a drinking glass. Water fills the bottom of the glass (representing your abdomen) first, and the top of the glass is filled with water last (representing your chest). Let's look at some useful tips for better breathing to improve your body's ability to preserve your telomeres and thus to slow or even stop aging.

Mouth Breathers Miss Out

The first (and last) time I ever took a Bikram Yoga class, I froze mid-move when the rather militant instructor singled me out—in front of the 40 other participants—by shouting over the loudspeaker:

"No, Ed! Bad!! You're breathing through the wrong holes!"

Even yoginis have bad days, I suppose, but she continued to massacre the endocannbinoids. She admonished the groaning class by saying, "You think I'm a bitch? You should ask my teen-age kids what they think of me!" I gave up the hope of finding my breathing catharsis that day and decided to not come back.

I still don't know which way was the non-Bikram way, but I do know that mouth breathing is not a good idea unless you are exercising vigorously, trying to dissipate heat, or scuba diving. In most situations, breathing through your mouth dries it out, which quickly causes poor oral hygiene, bad breath, and cavities. If you are breathing through your mouth, perhaps because of blocked nasal passages, you are not getting three crucial benefits of nose breathing: warming, humidifying, and filtering of particles.

Here's how your nose knows best:

- **Heating.** Breathing into the mucus-lined curvy shelves inside your nose slows the intake of air and provides the opportunity to warm up the air before it gets down to your lungs. Breathing in colder air than necessary wastes ATP to create heat and decreases efficiency of gas exchange by triggering airways and blood vessels in the lungs to constrict.

- **Humidifying.** Another benefit of breathing through your nose is its natural ability to humidify dry air. By humidifying the air, we prevent evaporative water loss from the mouth and lungs, which causes poor oral hygiene and impaired lung function respectively.

- **Filtering.** Mouth breathing puts a higher demand on your immune system because it allows particles like dust, pollen, airborne fungi, and even whole bugs into the air sacs of your lungs, where they are then only one or two cell widths away from directly entering your blood stream. These airborne critters, bad chemicals, and other crud place a burden on your immune cells by demanding that they respond by dissolving or ingesting them. If you inhale bacteria or particles that are too big to break up, the mucus we call phlegm will be excreted to coat them, and the cilia, or hairlike projections, in the air passages have to work extra hard to brush these invaders back up the chimney, as it were. It's a lot of work, and as we learned in Chapter 2, when you ask any organ to do a lot of work by replacing the cells, it ages the organ by replicative senescence. You are walking up the escalator, but the speed of the escalator has increased.

That's where nose breathing comes in. Your nasal passages provide the filter your mouth lacks. They are covered in fine hairs, nasal turbinates (curvy, bony outcroppings inside your skull), sinuses, and mucus to filter and deliver more purified air to your lungs.

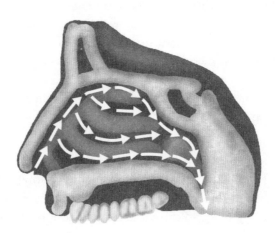

Anxious Breathing Is a Pain in the Neck

Do you have chronic neck and shoulder pain? One common reason might be that a depressed or anxious mood is influencing your breathing and posture.

When you are anxious, just like your poor ancestral caveman, who had to hide behind bushes from a tiger, you don't take full, loud belly breaths. Unconsciously, you take shallow sips of air using just the accessory muscles of breathing in your neck and shoulders. This kind of chronic, anxiety-caused breathing puts constant tension on your neck and ends up causing rock-hard and painfully tender muscle bands over and deep to the collar bone, about halfway between your breast plate and shoulder.

Neck breathing can also be caused or exacerbated by poor posture from sitting hunched or slouched at a desk for long periods of a time. When you are depressed, your posture tends to be collapsed. If your spine is not aligned correctly, the abdomen and chest are constricted and unable to expand properly, causing your inspiration to "cheat" by expanding up and triggering your neck muscles.

In another interplay of multiple TMTs, some of the most impactful and common problems we encounter with breathing occur while we sleep. Please refer to Chapter 6 to understand what could be the single most impactful thing you can do to improve health and longevity if you are one of the many people who suffer from sleep apnea (nonbreathing) and snoring.

So How Can We Breathe Ourselves Younger?

The simplest way that we can improve breathing is by maintaining good posture. This usually means maintaining erect posture and sitting up straight while seated. While sleeping, lying on your back with adequate spinal support is preferred, as being on your side creates some lateral compression of the rib cage. Many people have obstructive sleep apnea, so if that is a problem, correct it with a positive airway pressure machine.

BREATHING EXERCISES –
TEACHING YOURSELF HOW TO BREATHE

Once out of the womb and after taking his or her first breath, a baby naturally breathes properly. Unfortunately, babies aren't great instructors, so other than observing them, you can't learn a whole lot on the topic of breathing from infants. Plus, even if babies could teach a class, they wouldn't be able to help you out with breathing techniques to quell anxiety, for maximum performance during sports or exercise, or for overcoming fatigue, and more. Fortunately, there are many strategies you can use to optimize your breathing. Here are some techniques, but you should continuously experiment with getting to know how to breathe consciously.

1. "Square" Breathing to Improve Focus

This exercise is perfect to practice in the morning just after you wake up, or after a nap, when you're feeling rested and relaxed. Sit or lie down comfortably. Visualize a "square" of time with each side equaling 5 or 6 counts.

a. Relax your jaw, neck, and shoulders and place one hand on your chest and the other on your belly.

b. Inhale slowly through your nose and feel the hand on your belly rise and move outward. Focus on your belly rising and moving more than your chest.

c. Pause for 5 or 6 counts at the top of your inhale.

d. Exhale slowly for 5 or 6 counts. Feel your belly move inward as you press gently with the hand on your belly.

e. Pause for 5 or 6 counts at the bottom of your inhale to complete the square, then start again.

Feel free to experiment with changing the shape of the square to be more rectangular—if you want to pause for longer or shorter on certain "sides"—or even make it a trapezoid if you like! The magic comes from simply breathing consciously, not the specific shape or duration of the sides.

2. "4-7-8" Hold-Breath Technique to Relax

This technique is useful for calming general stress or anxiety.

a. Exhale completely through your mouth.

b. Close your mouth and inhale quietly and slowly through your noise for 4 seconds (count "One-one-thousand, two-one-thousand," and so on).

c. At the top of your inhale, hold your breath and count slowly to 7.

d. Exhale slowly and completely through your mouth, counting to 8.

This is one cycle; repeat three more times for a total of four breaths.

3. Paper-Bag Breathing to Counteract Hyperventilation

This is useful when experiencing moderate to severe anxiety or panic attacks, which are rare in most people but can be recognized by rapid, shallow hyperventilation and dizziness.

a. Hold a small paper bag over your mouth and nose.

b. Inhale slowly and naturally.

c. Exhale slowly and naturally.

Repeat for a total of 6 to 12 breaths, until your anxiety recedes.

4. Heart Breathing for Bliss

To generate happiness, sit in a quiet location and close your eyes. Place your left hand on your belly and your right hand on your heart. With each inhalation, imagine that your breath is flowing into and out of your heart. Summon a memory of a peaceful place and smile.

a. Inhale for 5 seconds, thinking, "Love is . . ."

b. Exhale for 5 seconds, thinking, ". . . everywhere."

Repeat for 15 to 20 seconds. You can make up any mantra you like: "I am . . . so free," or "My heart . . . is joyful."

5. Breath of Fire to Increase Energy

Instead of a cookie or coffee during your afternoon slump, try this strategy for a natural dose of invigorating awakening energy. It is a great way to greet the morning after meditation or to get energized for competition or a presentation.

a. Roll your shoulders back and down and sit comfortably, either cross-legged or in a chair with feet grounded.

b. Until you get proficient, you can place one or both of your hands lightly on your abdomen.

c. Exhale only through your nose with brief bursts of diaphragmatic elevations. The bursts should be 2 per second for 25 breaths.

d. Inhalation is passive.

e. Exhale it all out.

Repeat, while holding each of the following three locks:

- Lock one: Make a tight contraction of your pelvic floor (like you want to hold in a full bladder).

- Lock two: Pull your navel in and up.

- Lock three: Breathe into your chest and tuck your chin to your chest.

Congratulations! You are now on fire!

OTHER WAYS TO BREATHE YOUNG

While I'll come back to the following in the next chapters, I want you to have a sneak peak into the many ways that breathing affects and is affected by other activities and environments, and how you can optimize them to stay young.

Move for Better Breathing

How to breathe during cardio vs. strength training: Intermittent exercise challenges your lungs to take in more air, which exercises your lungs as well as your body and keeps your lungs, chest wall, and breathing muscles active, elastic, and strong. If you don't use it, you lose it. One caveat: if you don't exercise in healthy environments—such as running on a treadmill inside a coal mine—you won't do yourself any favors because the inflammation and toxins will provoke over copying of stem cells that shortens your telomeres.

During strength training: Don't hold your breath. Sometimes people have a tendency to hold their breath while exerting effort on a weight. This is dangerous. It is better to inhale as you stretch or load the muscles and to exhale as you contract or flex the muscles.

While doing cardio: Begin breathing in and out through your nose during your warm-up, and then when your intensity ramps up during the meat of your workout, you'll naturally breathe more through your nose and mouth. Let it happen—this gets more oxygen to your lungs and the rest of your body to meet the demands of your exercising body.

Correct Posture for Better Breathing

Poor posture affects your disposition, how you are perceived by others, and, most important, your breathing. You have to work harder to get breath into your lungs when your spine is collapsed or hunched while you stare at a computer screen or sit at a desk. When your posture is slouched, the accessory muscles of respiration in your neck have to work harder, which can create neck and shoulder pain, shallower breathing, and more anxiety. If your job requires hours at a desk, set a timer on your computer or phone to periodically remind you to sit up with your shoulders rolled back and down, and to keep both feet on the floor. You can also consider standing desks, kneeling chairs, or chairs with adjustable seat backs; just make sure you aren't slouched over and making breathing more difficult by collapsing your rib cage.

Mindful Breathing

Finally, we have the interesting notion of mindful breathing. Of all the tools we have to stay young and keep the telomeres in our stem cells healthy, conscious breathing is undoubtedly the most underutilized and yet potentially most powerful one. As we will discuss more in the next chapter, the mind, however consciously or unconsciously you choose to use it, can be a powerful ally or formidable enemy to healthy breathing, depending on how you use your consciousness. A good way to become relaxed is to meditate with mindful breathing. In the next chapter you'll learn such techniques.

Clean Air Acts

Ensure a healthy breathing environment. During many times of the year, plants and windy conditions release pollen and other allergens into the air that cause impaired breathing and allergic reactions. Keeping windows closed, wearing a filtration mask, and employing air filters may help, especially in your sleep chambers. It is important to change air filters in your home, car, and workplace. You should set a reminder for every six months at a minimum. You wouldn't keep doing laundry with a clogged lint trap, right? So why run the heat or air with a clogged and dirty filter? If there are conditions where fungus and mold could occur, it is imperative to find out and remediate them. If you are seeing multiple and serious problems with your energy, health, focus, or sinuses, there could be some mold hiding behind walls or in heating/air units that is constantly poisoning you. Humid or coastal areas, older houses, and leaky plumbing are certainly risk factors for a house infection with fungus or mold that could be harming you.

CONCLUSION

As we mentioned at the start of the chapter, breath is life. It follows that breathing is a powerful tool for bringing balance not only to your pH and blood gases, but also to your mood, your thoughts, and your optimal physiology. Whether you are singing, laughing, making love, meditating, or running, you are alive and breathing and you should be grateful for each breath that is keeping you balanced and on this side of the great divide.

The premise of this chapter is that you can become aware of and improve your breathing, resulting in healthier telomeres and a younger you. Luckily, most of the breathing you need to do is automatic, because such a critical function shouldn't be entrusted to beings who can misplace car keys and forget names. It might surprise you to know that I believe human consciousness can be viewed in the same way. Most thinking and its processing is automatic, although it is subject to some degree of voluntary control.

So in the next chapter, we'll explore a model of consciousness that my intuition led me to. We will explore how our thoughts, insofar as they can be controlled, can be a powerful ally to restoring balance and flow and therefore allowing our cells and their telomeres to be healthy and preserved.

As we build upon each new chapter, you may start to see a pattern: that each TMT affects the others. Are you more mindful because you're breathing well, or are you breathing well because you are more mindful? And what about breathing and sleeping or exercising? It gets confusing, I know. For the time being, we are only seeking knowledge. In time, intuition will lead us to wisdom and a more holistic view of the engine as more than just six separate cylinders.

Chapter 5

Your Mind

Seeing isn't believing. It works the other way around.

What is consciousness and how did our particular human flavor develop? At the outset, perhaps it was just a way to find our next meal without becoming someone else's. Not the strongest or fastest of creatures, our ancestors found that it was easier and more effective to look for food and stay safe with the help of others, so we developed symbolic language and more abstract thinking. The blessing and the curse of the human mind is that we are a species that is too good at creating stories and living outside the moment of real sensory perceptions and authentic feelings. So, to play nicely with each other, our cultures developed manners and obedience. As for the wayward mind, it still struggles with the ability to understand a variety of mind-sets, something that psychologists today refer to as "theory of mind."[1] This skill begins to function effectively around age five or six, when you are entering kindergarten. Theory of Mind is the notion that other people might have different points of view and motivations than your own. A paucity of this interpersonal connectedness is what we refer to as autism in children and narcissism in adults. In truth, empathy and the Theory of Mind are hardwired into human consciousness, because all consciousness is emotionally based and because we are heart-centered, social creatures.

Because we ultimately deploy all TMTs using our consciousness, the ability to have a well-rested, focused, and balanced mind-set will help us make optimal choices and maximize all the other TMT areas.

WHAT IS THE MIND'S PURPOSE?

To have the ability to understand each other, social animals, including humans, possess a key neurological device called "mirror neurons," a type of brain cell that has the ability to create a mental mirror of observed behavior as well as to allow for internal representations of another person's behavior. These mirror neurons are believed to help us empathize, understand, and "read" other people's minds. Monkey see, then monkey do—and then monkey wonders what made us both do that stupid thing. In studies that look at brain activity using functional magnetic resonance imaging (fMRI), scientists show that when one person watches a video of someone, the mind creates an internal and pseudo-experiential modeling of the observed experience. Whether it actually happens, you imagine it, or you see someone else do it—the same areas of your brain light up. These areas are your mirror neurons. You see someone smash his thumb with a hammer, you can almost feel it yourself—mirror neurons. You see a baby laughing in pure delight and you feel a surge of happiness—mirror neurons.[2, 3]

Interestingly, those mirror neurons are also what enable introspection, which is how you create a model for understanding yourself as a discrete person. It is noteworthy that mirror neurons are at the heart of both empathy for others and self-knowledge. One goal of this chapter is to leverage that bit of information to create a positive theory of mind about yourself that will better serve you—and your telomeres—to live a longer, happier, and healthier life.

In the 1990s, monkey studies led to the initial discovery of mirror neurons, but it wasn't until more recently that scientists detected that some people lack high-functioning mirror neurons (brain scans in these folks stay dark in response to another person's experience). In the extreme, we see this in the severely autistic person who has an almost entirely impaired ability to socially integrate. Not surprisingly, there is evidence that autism may be related to dysfunctional mirror neurons.[4]

To lack ego and a self may sound like elevated consciousness, but in practical terms, it looks more like the schizophrenic street person muttering expletives at you, inanimate objects, and himself. It might surprise you to know that we are all autistic, or internally preoccupied, to varying degrees; we just learn to suppress it, control it, and hide it.

For example, who hasn't experienced a surge of rage when someone cuts in front of you in line? You might find yourself mentally conjuring the idea that the offending party disrespects your age, gender, race, and so on. But then the offending ogre turns, smiles, and says, "Oh, did I just cut in front of you? I'm so sorry. I was lost in my own little world and I didn't see you—please go ahead of me." Our mirroring neurons suddenly have us smiling back. "Happens to me all the time," we might genially reply, before adding, "After you." What just happened? Motor neurons, manners, and millions of years of evolution just cost you your place in line. In contrast, clinical autism is a lucrative medical and business paradigm for psychiatrists and is defined by unusual difficulty with communication, relationships, and the nuances of linguistic subtext.

So here we are, social hominids on planet Earth, capable of astounding abstract thought and empathy, yet this fancy brain-power evolved on top of some other more primitive structures that often run things. Remember from the last chapter those brain-stem circuits that make it impossible to hold your breath too long or that make your heart race when danger is near? Those are older brain structures. Then, there are the newer, more nuanced abilities, such as mirror neurons, that allow you—but not your dog—to immediately recognize yourself in an *actual* mirror. Our minds are brilliant, but they can also be dangerous, constructing and believing some pretty bizarre and hurtful stories about others, and about our own selves. Ultimately, the tales you repeatedly tell yourself can make living a happy, long, and healthy life more difficult—and that brings us to the TeloMirror Tool that is your mind (this TMT also plays a central organizing role in how the other five TeloMirror Tools operate). So for the purposes of this book, the key to staying young is to harness the mind's ability and power to be balanced and present without being obsessive or reactive.

REALITY AND FREE WILL

Philosophers and scientists, who are just philosophers without a sense of history, have long debated consciousness. It is odd that even if a supreme and all-controlling god were to reveal itself to us, most humans would still believe in the following logical paradox: they have a material view of the world that somehow includes free will. Materialism states that the world is material and that spirit is not real. But if everything is just matter, then all your molecules should determine all your actions, right?

More accurately, materialism should actually be inverted: *it isn't that only the observable is real and to be believed, but rather that only what you already believe is observable and deemed real.*

For example, my son at the age of 12 told me that the *L* in the Staples logo was a staple, and I told him it wasn't. Then I looked at the logo with the intention of possibly seeing a staple there, and now I can't unsee it. But before my belief, it didn't exist. Quantum theory suggests that the act of observing, which is an act of consciousness, affects observable reality. If beliefs actively create reality, it follows that we can improve reality by modifying our beliefs. This book is about crafting optimal beliefs so you can change your reality on every level: from the telomere on up to the your life's purpose.

Medical research displays the same principle: only the observable is what is to be believed. One example is how most experts now agree that antioxidants promote cancer.[5] This may seem contradictory until you realize that doctors and the medical establishment don't make money on antioxidants; the bucks are in radiation and chemotherapy that antioxidants can sabotage (for more on antioxidants, see Chapter 9). On the other hand, evidence shows that chemotherapy doesn't improve outcomes in many cancer situations, but that proof is invisible because doctors profit from those treatments and feel good about doing something, even if it is objectively worse than doing nothing at all.[6] We all like to rationalize what benefits us.

In truth, much of scientific research perpetuates groupthink, is frequently unrepeatable, and oversimplifies truth in service of dogma. If you don't believe me, even Dr. Marcia Angell, a former editor turned whistleblower of the revered *New England Journal of Medicine*, confirms that much of what gets published is fudged, falsified, or dubious. This is just another example of not being able to see something you don't believe is there.[7]

Why discuss consciousness creating reality and the existence of free will at all in a book about telomeres? Because that is the human scale of experience in which we live. You can ponder gods, galaxies, and quantum states, but without free will, feelings, and morals, we are disconnected from everything that is meaningful in our human-scaled lives. As Alexander Pope wrote: "The proper study of mankind is man."

HOW DOES CONSCIOUSNESS WORK?

Throughout your life, your senses present your consciousness with information that is processed and assembled into data, schemes, and stories. As we will discuss in more detail later in this chapter, all this data is processed and potentially stored with the help of what I call *emotional meta tags*. This is the fundamental difference between human and artificial intelligence. A machine without emotion will treat all information as equal. But all your memories have emotional flavors and valences (or intensities) as well as stories attached to them; if they didn't, your limited storage space would soon be depleted. The mind is not as radically upgradable as are personal computers. We need to reuse our brains' hardware by actively creating, maintaining, and destroying neurons and the data, schemata, and stories they encode.

Disclaimer: My "emotional meta tag theory of consciousness" is a functional and empirical model of how the mind works. I am not a neuroscientist, and this theoretical construct is simply what I believe based on intuition and 50 years of experiencing my own consciousness. In website programming, a **meta tag** is a snippet of information about the information the viewer perceives on the web page. These tags aren't visible on the web page, but are part of the page's hidden code that includes information such as authorship, keywords, or even an explanation of why the page exists.

In our consciousness, it works the same way. For example, let's say that back when you were a child you had a dog, and let's say that one day your dog got out of the house. Imagine that you saw your dog across the street, and called to her, but just as she started toward you, she was struck by a car. You rushed to her, but it was too late, and she died in your arms. Now try to recall what you ate for lunch six days ago. One of these memories is much more emotionally charged than the other. Your dog dying is a memory that is meta-tagged with trauma, sadness, and guilt. If such an experience happened to you, it would likely change the way you process all stories surrounding dogs, cars, and traffic because of the strength of the emotional meta tag. It's unforgettable, whereas what you ate for lunch six days ago may never have lodged in your memory. To machine intelligence, on the other hand, "dead pet" and "Cobb salad" have the same emotional valence and meta-significance: none.

It is likely no accident that the limbic system in your brain (where the fight, freeze, or flight response is housed) controls emotions *and* regulates memory creation. Without emotions, we couldn't operate efficiently in our world. Not every person and every event can be of equal significance to us—emotions tell us what is important and what should be remembered. We would never make it down the street if we treated everything equally. Machines don't use emotions to color their information processing and that's why they are less adept at humor, obsession, passion, caution, and ennui.

The implication of what I'm saying is that, while we can't always control what happens to us in life, we can, to a great extent, choose what story, emotions, and importance we assign with meta tags. If we feel powerless, victimized, and threatened, this will degrade our health and wellness. Alternatively, if we find ways to feel empowered, supported, and grateful when experiencing life's challenges, we will grow and be more resilient and fulfilled.

The analogy of computer to brain offers many similarities that are useful when exploring how consciousness works, so let's draw out this analogy a bit more.

Let us consider your body's nervous system and your brain to be like the physical computer and its firmware. In contrast, your mind is your subjective experience of consciousness and is that user experience and software that determines what the computer accomplishes. But let us recognize that a bad user experience is also bad for your hardware by causing neglect of all six TMTs. Before we explore ways to "hack" our emotional meta tag system for better telomere health, let's take a moment to compare and contrast computers with how human brains and minds function.

HARDWARE, SOFTWARE, TASK MANAGER, AND THE USER

The Hardware and Motherboard

In computers, the *hardware* is made up of the physical components and circuitry of the computer's motherboard, and this is where the central processing unit (CPU) lives. The CPU handles what the computer is "thinking," but the motherboard also has alternative and parallel processors to handle graphics, communications, and other peripheral devices that run in the background.

By analogy, you believe that your consciousness is the answer to the question "What am I thinking?" But the reality is your consciousness is like the CPU and motherboard of a computer in that there are many processes that are "always on," helping to maintain homeostasis (staying the same or in balance) and perform surveillance (monitoring the environment). These other parallel processes include image processing, communications, introception (monitoring our body's condition), and a host of other bodily functions, such as breathing, heartbeat, and temperature regulation.

Our brains and nervous systems can be compared to the hardware of a computer, and they are made of cells that, except in the case of memory, don't often need replacement. Although neural stem cells and the brain's immune cells may age via telomere shortening from replicative senescence, this may not be as important a mechanism as direct damage for the majority of nerve cells, which are *post-mitotic*. Post-mitotic means nerve cells that are incapable of cell division, unlike the cells lining our intestines or generating our skin and hair, which divide and replicate all the time. You might say the brain was designed to run "for life," just as a computer's hardware is designed for the life of a computer, in a relatively solid state. Unfortunately, the "manufacturer" of human life span might not have predicted 100-plus years for many of us when we came off the assembly line.

Memory Storage and Retrieval

In computers, trivial memory is stored in the random access memory (RAM) for current usage by the CPU and disappears when the computer is turned off. The human version of trivial memory would be like the phone number of a pizza place in a town you will never visit again. It's unnecessary, so you don't remember it. A computer has a hard drive for storing more important information: this is permanent memory, and it is designed to hold on to valuable information long term. Similarly, in us humans, this is where you'd store the phone number of your standing local pizza delivery place, and this human hard drive is called declarative memory, or long-term memory.

The Software

A collection of meaningful and ordered routines that are summoned into the computer's "mind," or CPU, software is needed to perform routines for a specific purpose, such as organizing information into a spreadsheet or playing a movie. In human consciousness, this software function is referred to as *procedural memory*, and it includes habitual routines and behaviors such as "brushing my teeth" or "having patience with my kids." This software level is where we need to focus when it comes to making positive changes that will affect our beliefs and lengthen our telomeres. By upgrading our software to better versions, we can "hack" our own procedures—for example, by consciously choosing to focus on "counting 20 strokes as I brush my upper and lower teeth, front and back, inside and out, my tongue and gums, and my molars" or "intentionally saying something I love about my kids every morning." I'll come back to declarative and procedural memory in the next chapter, on sleep.

What's Running in Your Task Manager?

On a Windows computer, there is something known as the Task Manager that can tell you what software applications and system procedures are running simultaneously and in the background. Conveniently, you can hit CTRL-ALT-DEL and pull up a window that reveals everything that is at work to make your computer run. Similarly, if you could press your own CTRL-ALT-DEL and pull up the task manager of your brain right now, you might see programs such as peripheral vision, sounds to ignore, posture, muscles being used, temperature regulation, time awareness, hunger, bladder suppression, procrastination, regrets, fears, fantasies, and so on—what complicated creatures we are! These "programs" are not static like stored memory—they are flexible, purposeful, and logical, and for the most part, they are "always on" and running in the background.

So how you can exercise your mind to enhance your consciousness in a positive way? We can't turn off most of our body's processes, nor would we want to, but we can enhance presence and improve efficiency of our central tasks by making good choices attuned to whatever task we have at hand. Right now, that means that I need your full attention. Are you reading for maximum comprehension? That means that you are sitting comfortably, dressed for the current temperature, recently used the restroom, quenched your thirst, or had something to eat if you were hungry. I thank you in advance for your full attention.

When it comes to the last few items I mentioned in the human task manager list—regrets, fears, and fantasies—it is essential that they be muted for you to focus properly. As you read this book, your mind might turn to "fears of growing old," or maybe "fantasies of living to 200," or perhaps "regrets about picking up this book in the first place," but you are most likely able to put such thoughts on hold so you can pay attention to the content you are reading. Most thoughts don't need to be near the forefront of your mind, or even detectably running, while you're reading this book. If they are, you won't be able to fully use your mind.

That's why we need to learn to flow, mindfully breathe, and be in the present. That's the power in meditative and mindful practices. We strive to find the lesson and abundance in every moment, to calm and soothe erratic or irrational emotions, and to gain the grace to let go or make light of things that no longer serve us.

The User

In computer terms, the *user* is the person logged in to the computer. One computer can have multiple user accounts. So, on your computer, your partner and kids might each have their own log-ins, personalized desktops, and different software applications installed, and access totally different memories. In human terms, it is much less clear who the user is, but let's describe it as having three parts: the identity, the ego, and the soul.

What is identity? Your notion of identity might be described by discrete, subjective terms, such as "a 43-year-old conservative, white American teacher, born and raised in Chicago, and a mother of two school-age children." Of course, each of those terms can be refined and qualified *ad infinitum*. Maybe you identify yourself also in terms of your neighborhood, the clothes you wear, the car you drive, your job, your hometown, and so on. Identity tends to be superficial and is actually the easiest thing to change. Instead of thinking of yourself as a mother, you could view yourself as a parent. Instead of being of one specific race, you might identify with the human race.

What is the ego? *Ego* is Latin for "I," implying "I exist," and that is telling. "I exist" is not at all the same sentiment as, "I am part of life." The ego is a person's sense of self-importance and can be a bit of a dark force, because instead of uniting, it often focuses on differences, likes to set itself apart, and feeds its own importance. The ego is the roller-coaster ride of the human animal and it has a penchant for labeling everything as binary opposites: other people are either friends or foes, events are either beneficial or harmful, and so on.

Nevertheless, we came into existence to ride the roller coaster of ego. But ego is a restless seeker, and although it is a powerful ally for achievement and ambition, it conspires against bliss because it finds it hard to appreciate what it already thinks it possesses. Ego creates zero-sum games and conjures weird stories by whispering in your ear that you may need a better job, a bigger house, a flatter belly, and so on. The ego often uses many lesser demons to do its bidding. Maybe you've internalized the roles of "the jilted lover," "the cutthroat lawyer," or even "the victim of a traumatic childhood." Of note, in computer jargon, subroutines are also referred to as *daemons*. In us, our demons are hard to exorcise; in the very core of our weird user experience, we actually don't perceive them as malware, because they provide us excuses, plausible narratives, and a powerful energy. So instead of evicting them or labeling them, we can really only hope to defang them by making them feel like welcomed guests.

What are the temporary cures for ego running amok in your user experience? All the TeloMirror Tools, such as exercise, sleep, and meditation, can provide some temporary relief, but the real cure is found in your soul.

What is your soul? The soul is what remains when you cling less to identity and lessen attachment to the emotions that arise from ego-tripping. I define the soul as the pure light of consciousness that can and does organize into energy and matter and resonate with other souls. Unlike the inauthentic identity and the intemperate demons of ego, the soul can never be separate from the universe, because it is the very essence of the universe. The Sufi poet Rumi said, "You are not a drop in the ocean. You are the ocean in a drop." Perhaps the key to longevity may be to reconnect with the ocean as completely and frequently as possible. A drop can evaporate. But an ocean takes great effort to erase from existence.

I like what spiritual teacher Eckhart Tolle says of his greatest accomplishment: "to be able to just think of nothing." It is in that state of pure awareness, when all ego-demons are frozen and physical perceptions ignored, that we are able to simply exist in the eternal now.

So, how does consciousness work? You have a choice: you can either excessively nurture identity, become attached to the ego experience, and ignore your soul, which will accelerate telomere erosion; or you can clean out your "task manager" and upgrade your operating system so it understands how to surf the waves of life.

EGO-DEMONS: ANXIETY, RAGE, AND DEPRESSION—YOUR MIND'S WAR ZONES

What does it feel like to be a slave to unconscious fearful beliefs? Well, it might sound like one of the following:

- Anxiety: "If I am late to work again, I might lose my job." (A fear of the future.)

- Rage: "That person broke my heart." (A victim story of the past.)

- Depression: "I was short-tempered with my kids because I don't make enough money." (Internally directed anger around a disempowering story.)

What's the cure for obsession with the future, past, and perceived shortcomings? To be present with yourself, as strange as that sounds. You'll learn exercises to help with this in the next section, but before we explore them, let's try to understand both fear and relaxation pathways. Each plays important and complementary roles in maintaining homeostasis and keeping you in balance.

THE AUTONOMIC NERVOUS SYSTEM

A perpetually balancing and semi-antagonistic system known as the *autonomic nervous system* controls the global threat warning level system of your body. That means it impacts each and every cell and therefore determines their capacity to preserve and protect telomeres.

The autonomic nervous system is composed of the excitatory *sympathetic nervous system* and the relaxing *parasympathetic nervous system*. It would be tempting to call the former a "green light" and the latter a "red light," but like the ancient Taoist symbol of Yin and Yang demonstrates, each contains an essence of the opposing force, and for most systems to work properly, you actually need both sympathetic and parasympathetic systems to be cooperating. Lack of cooperation results in malfunction of systems such as heartbeat and breathing regulation, digestion, urination, and sexual function.

Yang, or the active and traditionally masculine principle, describes what people have referred to as "fight or flight." Yin, or the restorative and traditionally feminine principle, describes what people refer to as "rest and digest." Its nonurgent functions can be remembered by the acronym SLUDD (*salivation, lacrimation, urination, digestion,* and *defecation*), to which I'll come back.

EFFECTS

	SYMPATHETIC	PARASYMPATHETIC
EYE (PUPIL)	Dilation	Constriction
NASAL MUCOSA	Mucus reduction	Mucus increased
SALIVARY GLAND	Saliva reduction	Saliva increased
HEART	Rate increased	Rate decreased
ARTERIES	Constriction	Dilation
LUNG	Muscle relaxation	Muscle contraction
GASTROINTESTINAL	Decreased mobility	Increased mobility
LIVER	Glycogen to glucose increased	Glycogen synthesis
KIDNEY	Decreased urine	Increased urine
BLADDER	Contraction of sphincter	Relaxation of sphincter
SWEAT GLANDS	Sweating	No change

First, let's battle a tiger, which will illustrate how the autonomic nervous system handles danger versus security.

How Does the Autonomic Nervous System Function?

If a tiger were suddenly chasing you, your sympathetic nervous system would be triggered to cope with the clear and immediate danger. You'd be instantly wired with adrenaline and terror. When Mr. Tiger comes calling, there's no time for careful consideration—you need wide-open pupils, a forceful heart, higher blood pressure, wide-open lungs and oxygen supply, efficient cooling through sweating, high blood sugar, and adrenaline squirting out to increase fear and enhance memory. From an evolutionary perspective, this increased level of arousal means that if we survive this tiger attack, the next time we hear a growl and see a striped face, we will gain an extra step on the predatory tiger. This is an extreme example, but as explained by my emotional meta tag theory of consciousness, all learning, even nonlethal events and ideas, is encoded with emotions that were enabled by the autonomic responses. We often resent ourselves for being hung up on our inability to forgive today's petty insults or long-ago childhood traumas, like our dog being killed by a car after we called her, but the ability to encode danger and trauma serves to protect us; it was developed as a crucial survival mechanism.

Chilling Out

Let's imagine that you were on top of your game and you did manage to escape the tiger before it mauled you. Back at camp that evening, your Yin, or parasympathetic nervous system, would kick in. You would turn to activities that are restorative and relaxing now that the danger was gone. Now is the time for the Yin functions of SLUDD (*salivation, lacrimation, urination, digestion, and defecation*). To borrow a phrase from an old American beer commercial, "it's Miller [Beer] time." Perhaps someone gives you a nice scalp massage and you do some deep breathing to calm down. You sing songs about the legend of the tiger-slayer, stumble into the woods to enjoy a nice long pee and a bowel movement, and then retire to your tent to sleep it off.

You are in full Yin or parasympathetic mode. But if mama tiger should roar into your tent to rip you to shreds, you would instantly switch back to danger and survival mode. In contrast, if your drunken friend growled like a tiger while jumping into your tent, you might startle from sleep with a racing heart, but you would instantly recognize the fake threat and laugh or complain. Finally, if you viewed a body-cam video of yourself being attacked by the actual tiger, you would remain calm. The meta tagging tells you, "This is not really happening," and the exact same triggers are treated differently.

So the key to mastering the mind is to master the emotional meta-significance of all that you perceive. And here it is: deep within this chapter, we have found the gem we were searching for—*the key to mastering the mind is to master the emotional meta tagging of all that you perceive.*

By creating a safe space of mastery and detachment when needed, we can safely observe, participate resiliently, and reframe potential threats to maintain balance and flow. Whether facing a true threat, a joke, or simply a memory, we must always exercise semivoluntary control over our emotions. To paraphrase Reinhold Niebuhr's Serenity Prayer, cultivate the serenity to accept the things you can't change, the courage to change the things you can, and the wisdom to know the difference.

People's actions are their own karma, but if you don't resonate with them, they pass right through you. If we really perceive deeply, we see that most observed threats are trivial, impersonal, and fleeting, and as we grow older, we hopefully start to realize how little most people even think about us at all.

WHAT DOES TELOMERE SCIENCE SAY ABOUT THE MIND AND STRESS?

Remember that aging results primarily from low telomerase activity and critically short telomeres in your cells—one disease with a thousand faces. When you are stuck in the mind-set of fear, your mind and body are at constant battle with imagined tigers. The price is paid by your telomeres and the mechanism may be primarily hormonally driven.

Cortisol is a stress hormone that is activated when we feel danger. One of its main functions is to increase energy in the form of blood sugar (aka glucose). Cortisol also increases the sensitivity of your cells to the sympathetic nervous system that gets you primed for battle. This response originates in the central nervous system that signals the hypothalamus and pituitary gland to release hormones that will increase the adrenal gland secretions, a little yarmulke-like gland sitting on top of your kidney.

Since few actual modern life threats have the severity of a tiger attack, most of the "tigers" we perceive exist in the virtual reality of our minds; it follows that they can be interpreted according to our own intentional emotional meta-tagging. If we allow stress and the fearful ego-demons to dominate our lives, the long-term effects of bathing in excess, unopposed cortisol includes increased risk for diabetes, obesity, poor immune function, osteoporosis, infertility, stomach ulcers, and more. The adrenal glands become exhausted and our cortisol levels remain excessively low and unresponsive to actual threats.

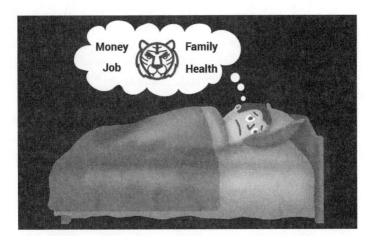

Consider the following research:

- Choi et al., in the journal *Brain, Behaviour, and Immunity* (2008), found that cortisol directly inhibits telomerase activity in our T cells, which are the cells that make up our immune system.

  Comment: This key insight from the UCLA School of Medicine provides the mechanism for understanding how stress ages us. Weaker immunity encourages chronic infections like CMV that age us and make it harder to eliminate damaged and potentially cancerous cells.[8]

- In a study published in the *Proceedings of the National Academy of Sciences*, researchers found that women who reported the highest levels of chronic stress had telomeres that were a decade shorter than those of women who reported the lowest levels of stress.

  Comment: Although the mechanisms are potentially complex, there is clear evidence that high stress is associated with shorter telomeres.[9]

- Practicing breathing and mindfulness techniques to decrease stress increases telomere length, according to research published in *The Lancet*. At the University of California–San Francisco, researchers found that when men followed a comprehensive plan including stress reduction techniques that incorporated breathing and mindfulness training, they decreased the age of their cells (as indicated by telomere-lengthening) by more than a decade. In addition to increasing telomere length, these strategies also boost serotonin and melatonin to increase relaxation, and reduce the stress hormone cortisol.

Comment: This study showed that telomere lengths are improved by only three months of mindfulness and relaxation training. Although both the intervention and control groups showed decreased telomerase activity after five years, the decrease was less in the mindful group.[10]

- Having close social ties may extend life. In an area of Costa Rica known as Nicoya, longer telomeres were associated with living communally with children, in all but extremely poor and extremely wealthy individuals.[11]

- When researchers at UCSF attempted to teach obese women mindful eating, body awareness, meditation, and yoga, two very interesting things happened. First, even women in the control group who didn't receive the treatment benefited, indicating that knowing they were part of a study made them somehow receive a powerful placebo effect. Secondly, both treated and untreated participants showed higher telomerase activity and improvements in stress, cortisol, dietary restraint, and food choices.

Comment: While the researchers would have obviously preferred to see drastic differences between treated and untreated groups, the bigger picture is even more empowering to us all. We are incredibly powerful in an intuitive way, even without the help of experts, and the ability to unlock the healing powers of telomerase and decrease stress, poor eating, and our own cortisol levels is accessible via that subconscious wisdom.[12]

- When a person is stressed out, it actually leads to a paradoxical effect on cortisol levels: adrenal glands become exhausted and cortisol levels are low. Chronic danger produces a paradoxically low cortisol level; the effect can be anxiety and depression, showing up as shorter telomeres, higher perceived stress, and even markers of inflammation, or C-reactive protein.

  Comment: This study ties it all together. High anxiety produces adrenal exhaustion, which leads to low telomerase activity. As discussed in Chapter 2, low telomerase activity will lead to telomere shortening, mutation, cell apoptosis, and the inflammation and oxidation that people misconstrue as the cause instead of the effect.[13]

HOW TO USE YOUR MIND TO STAY YOUNG

There are many ways for you to elevate telomerase activity by harnessing a positive and healing mind-set. This concept is nicely expressed with the Hawaiian word *lokahi*, which means to be in balance while still in flow. To block the Yang effects with blood pressure drugs or increase the Yin with heroin is not the best that we can do. It's like telling an autonomously driving car to step on the gas or the brakes. Just shut up and enjoy the ride. The *lokahi* state is to be open yet grounded, calm yet focused, and grateful and laughing in the present moment, no matter how your ego feels endangered.

Ultimately, we are trying to optimize function and make smooth transitions from conditions of excessive sympathetic or parasympathetic dominance.

Eight States of Consciousness Model

Of course, there is no best way of being conscious any more than there is a best color in the rainbow. I reject any one idea of optimal consciousness, or to put it more optimistically, I believe there are several fruitful paths to greater consciousness. This is good news because it means that you can put to use many flavors or colors that lead to higher states of awareness.

According to Hungarian-born psychologist Mihaly Csikszent-mihalyi, there are eight general essences of consciousness you can reach, depending on the degree of challenge and your skill level at doing some activity.[14] He suggests that people yearn for flow states because the emotions are harnessed in active performance and fully engaged learning. Perhaps this blissful state pleases us because we associate it with a temporary transcendence of our own demons.

You can see from the chart that if a task presents a high challenge but you have low skill to tackle it, it tends to create anxiety. For example, imagine dancing the tango in front of a room full of strangers when you don't know the steps. But if you were a lifelong professional dancer with high skill, you might find yourself in this same circumstance to be in a "flow" state of ecstasy.

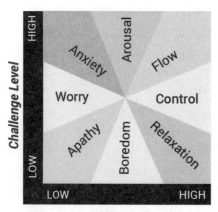

Skill Level

According to this scheme, a happier life would be achieved by deciding what skills you wished to pursue and then working to achieve mastery of them. Mastery allows us to experience relaxation with the easy ones, such as riding a bike, control with the moderate ones, such as making business calls, and flow with the hard ones, such as delivering a keynote address.

Extra Credit Question: What Is the Meaning of Life?

For most people, the meaning of life is a nearly constant meditation on the scarcity of money. As the chart shows us, these mental states occur when difficulty of survival is moderate to high and mastery is low. Since we cannot expect to be in an "upward spiral" if we are worried about money, I will only say that one of the greatest tools to keep your telomeres long is to live beneath your means, find ways to collaborate and share, and create as much financial independence as you can while maintaining joy and balance in your life.

"I promise you'll be happy, but even if you're not, there's more to life than that; don't ask me what." This wonderful line from *Fiddler on the Roof* asks us to sit uncomfortably with a big question. What is happiness, and should it be the central focus of a life well-lived? Buddhism teaches us that happiness is a fleeting emotion, ironically, in most cases, extinguished by actually attaining it. So, a better question is: How can we live lives that are fulfilling? That life would include three separate aspects of happiness: pleasure, immersion (or flow), and meaning.

We cannot be fulfilled with just pleasure and immersion (like being on drugs all the time) because there is little meaning in that. We cannot be happy with just immersion and meaning (like being an animal shelter euthanist) if we don't find the work pleasurable. And we won't be fulfilled with pleasure and meaning (like trying to make a baby) if we can't relax and go with the flow of the act of procreation. Pleasure + meaning + flow = fulfillment. It's like a three-legged stool: take away one leg and you lose stability.

Consider this quote:

> *Your beliefs become your thoughts,*
> *Your thoughts become your words,*
> *Your words become your actions,*
> *Your actions become your habits,*
> *Your habits become your values,*
> *Your values become your destiny.*
> *— Mahatma Gandhi*

This clearly expresses a logical argument. If we accept the series of statements and desire a fulfilling life, then it would be wise to start by examining our beliefs. And how do you examine your beliefs? You get conscious. You get quiet. You become aware!

Your beliefs are your mind's favorite, or most trusted, thoughts. Beliefs are learned, received, or fondly held ideas that are resistant to change. For some people, the existence of an omniscient and personal god or an afterlife might be a strong belief. Whatever serves you is fine. But if you want to make forward and upward progress in the arc of your life, you need to remodel and replace certain beliefs, which are the self-propagating malware or demons you foster. The seeds of these harmful beliefs may originate from how you felt parented, the reasons and remedies for feeling unsafe or unloved, or a notion that any aspect of your life is a conserved system rather than an open one.

Relax, You Were Never Fully Conscious and Certainly Not in Control

Whether we are sleeping, awake, in deep concentration, or in calm mediation, most of what passes for consciousness is made up mostly of unoriginal and automatic thinking that is only obliquely based in sensory perceptions. Consciousness is mostly a symbolic reality theme park that we conjure up for the amusement of our egos and their minor demons. In this wonderland, even our discernable thoughts are just the tips of old icebergs of belief that have hidden and trusted structures beneath. That's why we take comfort in brands, demographic checkboxes, our physical body, and language. Perhaps even more worrisome is that corporate media, using our collective beliefs, can manufacture reality, but that's a topic for another book.

On the other hand, if we existed in altered states of unadulterated pure consciousness and cosmic connection, like people having hallucinogenic drug experiences, living would be overwhelming, confusing, and quite dangerous. The pressure on your skin, the slightly different pitch of the engine noise of the car that drove by, the dryness of your right eye—the CPU of your mind would get overwhelmed by so many "signals" that it would struggle to find any order amid the chaos. That's why most of what we could potentially perceive is actively suppressed as background noise.

Think about how automatic thinking helps us. We can deftly control a two-ton car as an extension of our body. We obey traffic signals and avoid accidents and distracting strangers. We manage to drive all the way to work and not recall how we even got there, and yet our safety was not in question, despite our lack of awareness.

So, automated thinking is a good thing for getting through many of life's daily activities, but there is a downside. In fact, we are generally not very good judges of our own situations, because everything we think is filtered through the prisms of our unconscious reality mapping. For a billionaire who emerged from poverty, $10,000 won or lost in the stock market will not change his socioeconomic situation, but it still might trigger a sense of panic and danger akin to some major setback remembered from childhood, like the loss of a parent's job or the need to sell a home and move to the other side of town.

Of course, automatic thinking and the often crazy self-talk we can sometimes overhear is not random. They are the commerce of those demons of the ego that fight for primacy and obedience because we invite them to take up residence in our minds. It's these sorts of thoughts that cause chronic stress and anxiety, which accelerates the rate at which your telomeres shorten. The answer goes back to harnessing the power of your mind through heightened awareness and questioning your beliefs. Hard work, but it is worth it.

The Child Puts 2 and 2 Together and Gets 22

The most impactful beliefs that we have are laid down deep in our psyches during childhood and they color the way we experience the world. They form the roots of the thoughts, words, actions, habits, values, and destiny that ensue.

For that reason, it is important to at least attempt to deconstruct them in an attempt to harness their power and tame any dysfunctional effect they may have upon our experience. It is these thoughts that inform our self-image, our ways of relating to others, and self-talk.

If a child had an abusive and alcoholic parent, she might internalize the idea that her actions, or even her core identity, were producing the traumatic actions of the parents. It is also likely that a toxic parent fosters false beliefs in his child because he also received similar treatment from an older generation of toxic parenting. The voices in your head may simply be the voices in your grandparents' grandparents' heads.

In contrast, a child who is told he or she is special and always receives unearned praise and exceptional treatment may become narcissistic and poorly integrated into society. Such children internalize the narrative that they are very special, and when the world doesn't reward their innate superiority with favors but instead requests grades, performance, time, and building of relationships, they fail.

Unless and until a person awakens to the awareness that his or her parents and life partners may have helped create false beliefs about him- or herself, this individual will suffer. He or she may even seek out relationships that recapitulate this dysfunctional relationship in a vain attempt to "fix" what seemed so broken with this important relationship.

All beings must work to exorcise these false associations constructed while they only possessed the faculties of a self-centered and sensitive child. Thoughts like "If I stand up for myself, I will be attacked" or "I'm so bad that people I love abandon me" can echo for an entire lifetime if people don't examine and deconstruct those beliefs in a more holistic and positive context.

HOW TO IMPROVE YOUR MINDFULNESS

There are no literal tigers in your life. It is all in your head. That's not to say you don't have to pay your bills and maintain healthy relationships. All things considered, if we nurture negative thinking patterns we will manifest counterproductive beliefs and behaviors and cause a downward spiral, allowing our telomeres to shorten. Bad thoughts lead to impaired breathing, insomnia, depression, disinterest in exercise, emotional overeating, and so on. In contrast, an upward spiral results when beliefs are reframed by practicing positive thinking. Let's discuss the ways we can learn about, then accept, and finally harness the demons running in the background of our consciousness.

Here are some of my favorite ways to encourage a telomere and telomerase fostering mind:

TMT Mind-Hack #1: The Quick Fix Is Just to Breathe

Your mind is the mediator and mitigator of all the other TMTs. If you haven't yet mastered the ability to be in the present moment, then focusing on breathing always brings you back. Close your eyes as you sit or lie down somewhere quiet or put on headphones. Eyes open, eyes closed, with or without holding your breath . . . it is all good as long as you are consciously breathing into your abdomen. For more ideas about mindful breathing, turn back to the exercises in the last chapter.

TMT Mind-Hack #2: Laughter Is an Orgasm of the Soul

At my 25th college reunion, I saw a classmate who shockingly hadn't aged a day. One peculiarity of her personality was that she audibly laughed at the end of nearly every sentence. This habit may have given her extremely good respiration, relaxation, endocannabinoid levels, and other healing powers. Laughter is working two TMTs at once: breathing and consciousness. Whereas the storytelling of our dramatic ego wants to suffocate in the seriousness of everything, the spirit of laughter says, "Let go. All is absurd and so at least enjoy that." There is a good reason they call it the "best medicine." I recommend keeping a brief comedy skit that always makes you laugh on your smart phone or computer. Search the Internet for videos of laughing babies, goats yelling like humans (yep, it's a thing), or old *SNL* skits that tickle your fancy. When in doubt, laugh it out.

TMT Mind-Hack #3: Meditation Is Eavesdropping on the Demon Chatter

If you want your telomeres to mirror positive tendencies, then you need to know how your mind actually operates to generate negative ones—meditation is the key that unlocks the mind's door. Meditation can be compared to running a disk defragmenter because it frees up drive space and helps your mind to run better, faster, and more efficiently. The current Dalai Lama says sleep is the best meditation, but if you aren't able to nap, then meditate. Meditating brings harmful demons to the surface where they can be uninstalled. At first, meditation can seem like a waste of time. You are just sitting quietly, upright, with your eyes closed and fingertips touching, with an intention of concentrating on your breathing. And then your mind goes into hyperdrive, playing all sorts of noise and chatter. You'll hear voices from your parents, friends, and other significant relationships past and present. A lot of people think that they are failing to meditate when this happens, but this is all just a part of meditation. There are countless ways to meditate, and I encourage you to experiment to find what works best for you. To get started, try this simple meditation:

Sit comfortably and quietly in a place you won't be disturbed. Set a timer for five minutes. Close your eyes and bring your attention to your breath. Don't try to change your breath in any way, just observe your inhalations and exhalations. Notice how your breath flows in and out, noticing how your body feels. When thoughts arise, and they will, think of them as clouds in the sky passing overhead. When you notice that your mind has drifted from your breath, smile to yourself, and gently bring your attention back to your breath. Continue to feel the air entering your nose, imagine following the breath down into your diaphragm, and feel as you exhale, blowing out through your mouth.

Over time, using meditation regularly, you can distance yourself from destructive and defeating self-talk and even create "antidote mantras" to negate them (the next Mind-Hack explores these mantras in more detail). Try the above meditation, but add variation by focusing on sounds instead of your breath, or by repeating a positive word such as *peace* or *love*. There are also great meditation apps, such as Insight Timer, Simply Being, and Mindfulness, that you can use just about anywhere.

TMT Mind-Hack #4: Use C.A.R.E. to Refurbish Those Old Beliefs

You help care for "the user" (your mind) through better identity hygiene. What is identity hygiene? Let's use the mnemonic of **C.A.R.E.** to remind us to Clear, Audit, Reframe, and Enjoy. Here's how it works: Whenever you have a situation that hooks you—anything that triggers, makes you see red, or strikes fear or sadness—you can apply this acronym letter by letter to keep your mind calm, cool, and collected—and functioning fully. Let's use driving in your car as a common example as we move through the following steps.

Clear the clutter that you identify with in your physical, emotional, spiritual, professional, and social life. You might be surprised to know how infrequently others think about you, so you can also expend less energy on what you should be looking like, feeling, believing, and doing. Let's say you are stuck in traffic and late for an important business meeting, and you feel your anxiety strike. You might find yourself thinking, "That's it, I'm about to be fired." To clear the chatter, turn your focus on to your breath and those thoughts will pass.

Audit the voices: listen to the demons in your head that say things like "I'm out of control." Once you find those demons, create an antidote mantra and attach it to breathing like so: Inhale while thinking, "I am," exhale while thinking, "powerful." You can also create positive self-talk mantras as well. Look in the mirror, stand up straight, smile, and say, "I choose to be happy in this moment."

Reframe: The most powerful thing you can probably do is a trick we will call **reframing** with gratitude. Whenever something elicits a powerful negative emotion, attempt to defuse it by reframing it with gratitude. People's negative actions and emotions are their karma, and like any unwanted gift, you can decline to accept them. When someone tailgates you and flips you the bird, you might consider, "I am grateful that I was reminded to keep up with traffic and to be mindful of those behind me." You will get two additional benefits from the emotional judo trick. You will have fewer things emotionally meta tagged to clutter your consciousness and encode as memories and dreams. Also, you will have a valuable tool of self-discovery, as most things that make us angry in others often reflect things that we don't like about ourselves. What we resist persists. Reframing leads to enhanced compassion for others and ourselves.

Enjoy: Enjoyment comes when you align yourself with abundance and compassion of living. You are living "IN JOY" when you EN-JOY. Seeking the enjoyment of each moment will bring better focus, attract more luck and better people, and reveal your true destiny, because your intuitive feelings are seldom wrong. Synchronicities will abound when you are not locked in some crazy story told by inner demons. Follow your bliss in every moment.

To be free of dysfunctional beliefs, seek to always C.A.R.E.— clear, audit, reframe, and enjoy.

What Does Healing Catharsis Feel Like?

Twice, I have had rapid and efficient feelings of emotional catharsis. Once was as a result of "energy healing" and the other was from a heavy "gong bath" of sound during a yoga class. Each day, on a smaller scale during my hot yoga classes, I also get to exorcise while I exercise from deep breathing and movement with other conscious yogis and yoginis. Sometimes a really great movie can also elicit this catharsis—that is when you recognize what an exorcism truly is.

It can come with trembling, strong emotions and vivid depersonalization, electric sensations, and even laughter. The best way I can explain it would be that the crazy thoughts that you once identified with become as clear as if you were to shine a flashlight on a kid in a goblin costume in a haunted house. They dust themselves off and you may offer them a hug or a handshake as they politely escort themselves out of your psyche. They may revisit from time to time, but the experience of seeing and distancing yourself from certain dysfunctional and ultimately false beliefs is profound and the basis of true healing.

CONCLUSION

I believe we are all computers that use emotions, not silicon chips, to create stories and beliefs. Those stories and beliefs make up your experience of life and powerfully impact those around you. Thankfully, as with breathing, we can discover ways to exert semivoluntary control over how we meta tag information. Did you ever stop and think that perhaps the reason we encounter the same darn problems over and over again is because like the Phil Connors character from the movie *Groundhog Day*, we haven't actually learned the lessons we need to move on?

The simple statement "Wherever you go, there you are" can be understood as a Yogi Berra-esque aphorism, but it can also be expanded out like a fractal image to explain the suffering inherent in the human condition. If the roof leaks, you move, stop the drip, or open an umbrella. You wouldn't just sit there and endure it, right? Yet often we just wallow in unpleasant situations when we could transform our reactions and thereby transcend. More often than not, there are probably some hidden benefits from wallowing that you could pay a therapist thousands to help you discover. Or you could just look deeply and honestly within.

From the mundane daily grind: Do you hate rush hour traffic? Well, what if you left for work 25 minutes earlier? Would you get there an hour earlier and be able to go the gym and even shower?

Bad relationships? Perhaps you partner with the same type of codependent person that brings out the worst in you? By clearing the clutter and auditing the voices, you might uncover the weirdness about relationships that you might have learned as a child so that you can move forward.

Cosmically, perhaps you reincarnated as a stressed-out human because a few lives back, you were a dolphin that refused to play with others? Maybe you are not even going in the right direction, reincarnation wise! Perhaps it is time to master your consciousness before you backslide into even less conscious form?

So, wherever you go, there you are! From your entire existence, down to each millisecond of consciousness. You are always in the presence of your own mind, but are you truly present with your emotions and friendly with the demons that are conjuring reality on your behalf? Are you able to transcend your perceived problems by reframing with gratitude? Don't abandon yourself or medicate away your feelings. Feelings are trying to guide you to what needs to happen in order to evolve and live a more blissful life. What you hate is ultimately what you need to heal.

Seek compassion for yourself and forgive everyone everything. You can begin to do this by making regular use of the four Mind-Hacks in this chapter. Holding on to trauma and old grudges can fill you with dark energy, and the cost to your health and happiness is too great. Instead, seek to accept that everyone is on his or her own journeys and that your job is to be the best version of yourself, not to coerce others into what you perceive as wisdom and righteousness.

I was being facetious when I said consciousness is just a means to find the next meal. Consciousness is the essence of existence, so relish it! To love, to feel wonder and beauty, to laugh at the pathos and absurdity of it all—it is a great honor to be human. When you surrender to that truth, you will appreciate the miracles that are omnipresent in what once seemed a predictable and pointless "Groundhog life." Remember how Phil Connors dreaded waking up to the same serial day? Sleep was the frontier that he needed to cross, and one magic morning he awoke and it was a brand new day. We do the same, but we try to trick ourselves into believing each day is just a little different but mostly the same.

Sleep is another "undiscovered country" that Hamlet alluded to in his soliloquy about life and suicide. Sleeping is a little death, and that is why Saint Paul said, "I die daily." Functionally, sleeping serves as a sort of Etch-a-Sketch shake up and a nightly C.A.R.E. routine. Our identities are CLEARED and allowed to become fluid and chaotic. We observe and AUDIT the demons as they rearrange furniture in the haunted houses of our psyches. But are we maximizing bliss by REFRAMING with gratitude? These are the skills that we will master in the next chapter about sleep, one of the most crucial TeloMirror Tools that we have. To ENJOY sleep enables us to have healthier and longer lives while we are awake and keeps all the cylinders firing together to keep the telomeres long and healthy.

Chapter 6

Your Sleep

This day seemed a pointless
and regrettable interruption of sleep.

I once heard my intensely driven mother say she wished she didn't have to sleep at all, as if nearly a quarter of her life was being wasted. Sadly, this sentiment is a common belief and shows a lack of understanding regarding the primacy of sleep. Even sharks that need to continually swim to oxygenate their gills have evolved to sleep one cerebral hemisphere at a time.

THE PRIMACY AND PURPOSE OF SLEEP

(Or, Why "I'll sleep when I'm dead" is a dangerous life motto)

Wishing for the ability to live without sleep is like saying, "I wish no one cleaned the office at night so we could work around the clock shifts," or "Wouldn't it be great if we could just eat and never have to poop!"

The cleaning analogy is right on point in that sleep is when the brain's immune system literally takes out the trash. This so-called "glymphatic system," or glial lymphatic system, is defined as a waste clearance pathway that not only clears away rubbish, but also renourishes the entire central nervous system with glucose, fats, proteins, and more. There are multiple studies suggesting that poor sleep precedes Alzheimer's disease, so the question is, is that association causal? A University of Rochester study of anesthetized mice showed that while in deep slow wave sleep, their brains expanded to have more fluid space between cells (interstitial fluid) and enhanced the clearance of Beta amyloid (a protein that accumulates in Alzheimer's disease).[1]

The pooping analogy is also apt. During the day, we take in the "food" of experiences, memories, and the stories we construct around them. At night, we release the "poop" of what didn't move us or what wasn't deemed useful. This process serves to preserve emotionally meta-tagged life experiences into stories, beliefs, and skills—and to let go of useless or cluttering information.

But sleeping is not only a time of brain cleaning and psychic maintenance; it is also when the body most efficiently heals itself. During slow wave sleep, growth hormone peaks and there is massive cell replication. Think about the busy highways where you live. They don't repair the roads on Monday morning, right? They do it Sunday evening when the roads are not actively used. Just so, the nighttime is the right time to regrow telomeres, repair or clear damaged cells, and refresh the mind.[2, 3]

So, Why Do Rats Die if They Are Sleep Deprived?

In a rather morbid study, it was established that rats die when deprived of sleep for extended periods of time. In 1989, University of Chicago researchers subjected 10 unfortunate rats to total sleep deprivation. All the rodents in the study were dead after 32 days. The researchers could find no specific cause of death, but all sleep deprived rats showed ragged appearances, lesions on their tails and paws, and weight loss in spite of increased food intake. Control rats that were allowed to sleep stayed healthy. Similarly dark studies have been done on pigeons with comparable outcomes.[4]

While no humans are known to have died from staying awake for extensive periods of time (most human studies of sleep deprivation are just two to three days in duration), research does show that sleep deprivation in humans is associated with mental and mood problems, immune dysfunction, diabetes, cardiovascular disease, shorter life spans, and more.[5, 6]

Of course you don't really need scientific studies to tell you that lack of sleep makes you feel cruddy in every possible way. I'm sure you can attest to feeling lethargic, unfocused, foggy, fatigued, and irritable. These are the subjective manifestations of the failure to repair and restore that occurs in all cells when you are sleep deprived. What is the opposite of these run down, ragged symptoms? The way you feel after getting great sleep.

Although sleep deprivation subjectively feels reversed after one good night, we might be fooling ourselves. Perhaps we can store up and deplete sleep in the form of telomere lengthening? You are sprinting back up the escalator of telomere attrition when you sleep. In contrast, if you are chronically sleep deprived, you are heading for the telomere basement because normal telomere shortening is not being reversed during the hours that you are skipping rest.

HOW IT WORKS: THE BASIC MECHANICS OF SLEEP

What is sleep? Sleep is described as a state of diminished conscious awareness in which the nervous system is relatively inactive, the eyes are closed, the postural muscles are relaxed, and sensory stimuli are mostly ignored. In a way, sleep is like shifting to a different gear.

In Chapter 5, we discussed the fact that, even in waking life, there are various degrees of awareness, and filtering of thoughts and ideas, that depend on the various demons running in our consciousness. As we sleep, we are still capable of sensing and responding to changes in the environment, but there is a downshifting of sorts that enables a myriad of mysterious repair and maintenance programs to run. Another way to see this is from an Eastern point of view: your day uses your yang energy for the action of your ego and bodies, while the night uses your yin energy for recovery and restoration of your mind and body.

From outside observation, your slumbering body might appear relatively immobile, but on a cellular level your mind and body are involved in frantic metabolic activity including cellular copying and increased clearance of waste products when compared to non-sleep time. Sleep is a time of massive anabolic (cellular growth) changes in your body, which explains why human growth hormone peaks during the early part of the night.

The first part of your sleep phase is characterized by slow wave and deeper sleep, and it's also when declarative memory (long-term memory) is formed by neurogenesis (new brain cell creation).[7] Like maintaining a computer hard drive, the early, slow wave, and deeper sleep provides a nightly "defragmentation" of your mind and writes new memories by actually creating thousands of new brain cells.

Later in the evening, rapid eye movement (REM) sleep makes sense of memories and meanings by constructing stories and meaning around them. In this phase, we are upgrading the software versions in our minds. Without both types of sleep, we become dysfunctional both because our memories and mind-set are impaired. Sleep deprivation and dysfunction, which is tied to insomnia, mood disorders, and addiction, impairs learning and neural plasticity. Lack of sleep is how we stay stuck in static and flawed narratives about ourselves and the world; it is how the demons lead us to insomnia, legal and illegal drug use, mood disorders, and even suicidal ideation.

In the "Dunning-Kruger effect," a phenomenon named for researchers Dunning and Kruger, individuals over- and underestimate their intelligence and competence.[8] In a series of studies, the researchers found that those with less competence rated themselves as high and those with high competence rated themselves as low. Sleep deprivation is clearly linked to lower cognitive ability, which means that the sleep-deprived (who make up an estimated

35 percent of the population, according to the CDC[9]), would more likely be affected by a sort of Dunning-Kruger effect with regard to sleep self-evaluation. They are so impaired by sleep deprivation that they can't even recognize that they are sleep deprived.

A True Genius Never Sleeps?

Leonardo da Vinci reportedly took 20-minute naps every four hours, and Nicola Tesla claims to have never slept more than two hours a day. You've probably heard of high achievers who boast of thriving on six or less hours of sleep. This popular folk hero is the highly successful, but socially awkward tech CEO who proudly self-identifies with what has been fashionably labeled Asperger's syndrome. This type used to be just called "nerdy," but is now said to be "on the spectrum" of pervasive developmental disorders (PDD). Such men, and they are usually men, are disciplined, often in good physical shape, and high achieving. However, if you know or have known someone like this, perhaps you have also noted a certain dearth of irony, humor, and social flexibility in them. Perhaps this competence and ability for social engagement is missing because of the lack of adequate sleep?

Most humans who live concrete lives of facts and figures without regard to the complexities of fuzzy human relations don't actually run billion dollar companies; they often struggle for workplace recognition, have rocky familial relationships, and have difficulty maintaining casual friendships. Maybe social skills and emotional intelligence would be enhanced by more hours of sleep every night?

Is Oversleeping a Sign of Depression or an Attempt at Healing?

A standard psychiatric interpretation of hypersomnia (sleeping too many hours or feeling too drowsy) is that it is a common sign of depression. I would like to agree, but I find that no matter what is going on in my real life, if I sleep extra hours, I awaken in a good mood and if I sleep the "normal" amount of time, I am cranky. What if excess sleep is not a sign but rather an adaptation to ameliorate stress? Just as an injured animal may sleep all day, the person in crisis may be utilizing longer periods of sleep to repair the damage of life stress. If you allow those demons to reboot too early after a mere six to eight hours, they might just continue whispering those not-so-sweet nothings in your mind's ear.

There is a biological truism that says "[developmental] ontogeny recapitulates phylogeny." This means that as an embryo develops, its sequential forms resemble the stages of species evolution, such as a shared tadpole or amphibian stage. If we take note of the order of sleep ontogeny described below, we see that the physical body heals first, then the declarative memory of brain cell regeneration and data storage takes place. Finally, the procedural memory or software is upgraded as would be required by story-telling social animals. But what if there is a future evolution toward interconnected and compassionate humans? Perhaps sleeping "too much" is just our way of accessing the phylogenetic benefits that have yet to take place in our human evolution? Instead of feeling animosity and helplessness, extra sleep transports me to a future consciousness where I can gratefully reframe the "slings and arrows of outrageous fortune" into spitballs and Nerf arrows of an absurd yet manageable comedy.

This is not to suggest that you should ignore oversleeping when it is accompanied by other signs of major depression: suicidal ideation, guilt, depressed mood, lack of enjoyment, inability to concentrate, and changes in appetite. You may need to consult a psychiatrist if you experience several of these symptoms. But if a nap or a few hours extra of sleep can keep you off medication and in a good mood, perhaps it is worth a try first.

OPTIMAL FUNCTIONING: THERE IS SUCH A THING AS OBJECTIVELY GOOD SLEEP

While it may be hard to achieve at times, good sleep is not hard to describe. Optimal sleep patterns for most adults can be described by six complete and highly structured 90-minute voyages into altered consciousness that you take in the comfort of your own comfortable, safe, and blissfully dark bedroom. Most people don't realize that they often awaken between 90-minute sleep cycles. Highly sensitive brainwave, breathing, and eye movement measurements confirm this. Like the three-second pause between songs on the radio, you don't normally recognize the brief awakenings between sleep cycles unless your partner is snoring, it is loud, you need to use the bathroom, or you are too cold or hot.

These brief awakenings happen every 90 minutes throughout your night, and indeed the entire aggregate of sleep duration naturally organizes into multiples of 90 minutes unless you are living by the alarm clock. That means that if you sleep just 4.5 hours you go through three cycles, six hours gives you four cycles, seven and a half provides five cycles, and eight and a half hours confers six cycles. (Note: after the sixth cycle of sleep and onward cycles tend to shorten to 60 minutes' duration.)

Ideally those eight and a half hours are free from difficulty keeping an open airway (snoring and apnea), anxiety about safety (real or psychic tigers), not more than one trip to void your bladder, and in most cases, should not require you to eat, defecate, or answer e-mails. I've mentioned the early cycles of sleep already in this chapter; let's take a deeper look at all the cycles of sleep and how they differ in structure and function.

Normal Sleep Cycles and Their Stages and Architecture

As a point of reference, keep in mind that normal brain chatter operates at the beta brain wave frequency of about 15 to 40 cycles per second or hertz (1 hertz equals 1 cycle per second; any cycling rate is known as hertz or Hz) During times of high-level insight or intuition we can achieve frequencies above 40 Hz, called gamma brain waves.

Sleep architecture is easy to document by monitoring brain waves and body and eye movements that are observed during each sleep stage. During each 90-minute cycle of sleep you enter and exit several possible types of modes or stages classified into two general classes: rapid eye movement (REM) and non-REM.

Below is a figure of an electroencephalogram (EEG) legend that shows the typical brain waves exhibited during each sleep phase or cycle.

Brain Waves during Sleep

When we are awake, the electrical activity measured by scalp electrodes above the brain is the rapid beta form mentioned above. During each of the stages of sleep, patterns emerge corresponding to mysterious but likely practical subroutines that your central nervous system is carrying out. Let us take a moment to characterize the stages by the EEG patterns and other phenomena that are measured and experienced in each phase.

Non-REM Stage 1 (about 10 Percent of Total Sleep)

Alpha wave or eyes-closed relaxation (8 to 13 Hz) is the light sleep stage that the brain enters at the start of a sleep cycle or exits at the end of a sleep cycle. It is like the airlock you pass through before and after a trip outside your submarine or spaceship. It is during this drowsy state during that people have twitches and hallucinations (sights and sounds that are not present in the outside world). During this transition, the mind is slowing from 8 to 13 cycles/sec or Hz to 4 to 7 Hz or the theta brain wave state. There is moderate loss of muscle tone and conscious awareness during this stage.

HUMAN SLEEP STAGES

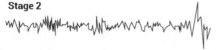

Awake

Drowsy

Stage 1

Stage 2

Delta Sleep

REM Sleep

Non-REM Stage 2 (Nearly Half of Total Sleep Time)

Theta waves (4 to 7 Hz), sleep spindles, and K-complexes are a phase characterized by deeper sleep, during which soft, slow theta brain waves are observed with brief interruptions of two forms of higher frequency waves. The first type is brief and tight, resembling a spindle on the EEG. The second type of wave is larger and more sustained and called a K-complex.

Research shows that both K-complexes and sleep spindles may have a role in creating declarative memory during the earlier sleep cycles of the night. This is when the facts are put to tracks. The new brain cells and their neural pathways are being fired up for the first time like lighters during a slow ballad at a rock concert.

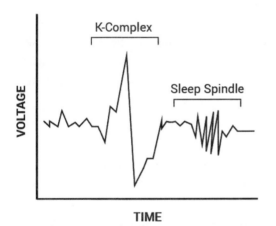

It's interesting to note that the theta brain wave pattern is what trained monks can enter during meditation. Some people believe this is a common wavelength for telepathy, cosmic consciousness, or the world soul, if you believe in any of that stuff. Muscle tone and conscious awareness of the environment are greatly diminished.

Non-REM Stage 3 (20 Percent of Total Sleep in Adults)

Delta waves of high voltage and low frequency (<2 Hz). This stage is dominated by *slow-wave sleep* (SWS) or very deep restorative sleep. The sleeper is hard to awaken and the body is essentially paralyzed. It is during this phase that parasomnias like sleepwalking, bedwetting, and night terrors can occur, and if awoken, the sleeper will be very disoriented. During this deep sleep, the cells are rapidly copying.

REM Stage (20 Percent of Total Sleep)

REM Sleep (8 to 13 Hz). During this phase, the sleeper is hard to awaken, the eyes move rapidly, and breathing and heart rate are deregulated. In other stages, breathing, heart rate, and blood pressure are reduced.

It may be that the full autonomic, emotional meta-tag verisimilitude of virtually real dreaming is required to form emotional imprints on the dream storytelling of procedural memory. Remember, this type of memory is created for common routines or habits such as "brushing my teeth," but also is involved in complex stories like "being a good spouse." During REM sleep, the brain waves are rapid and the mind is actually creating its own virtual reality simulation.

Though the sleeper is unconscious, REM sleep is a near-wakeful state of consciousness and occurs near the beginning or end of the night's later 90-minute cycles, unlike the delta slow wave sleep that is typical of the earlier cycles. That means that when you cut your sleep short, your REM sleep is being sacrificed.

Brief Awakenings

Once you reach the end of each 90-minute cycle, you wake briefly even if you are unaware of it, then head down your next cycle.

Now that you understand the different stages of sleep, the hypnogram on the facing page can be understood.

HYPNOGRAM

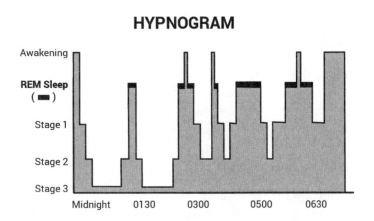

As you can see from the hypnogram, normal sleeping shows three general patterns.

1. Earlier Sleep Is Dominated by Theta Waves and Slow Wave Sleep

At the nadir of your first two 90-minute cycles, an EEG would show you spending most of the time in Type 2 NREM (theta waves) and Type 3 NREM (delta waves) sleep. This coincides with your growth hormone release, physical and cellular repair, and formation of declarative memory via neurogenesis. Later in the night, this deeper type of sleep typically does not occur.

2. Stage 1 Is Just a Transitional State

Secondly, we see that drowsiness (Stage 1 NREM) is a transitional stage, like the first 10 feet of a scuba dive, either ascending or descending. Stage 1 alpha wave sleep is merely a path down into deeper Stage 2 NREM or back up to lighter REM sleep or wakefulness. It can be recognized by the twitches seen in the sleeper.

3. REM Sleep Dominates Later Cycles

Third and finally, most of our time in later sleep cycles is spent in REM sleep. Perhaps this represents an evolutionary prioritization of physical repair and declarative memory (making concrete and long-term memories) over higher learning and emotional equilibrium during times of limited sleep. As mentioned in the section on hypersomnolence, it's also plausible that the ontogeny of sleep architecture recapitulates sleep phylogeny as well (the order of expression is last because it was the latest to develop).

Declarative versus Procedural Memory

It is during the earlier sleep cycles that the declarative memories (faces, numbers, names) of the day that have been tagged with emotional significance are saved from our RAM (random access memory) of short-term mundane memories into more semipermanent neural "hard drives" with the help of something called prions (or proteins that shape mimic other proteins) and the formation of new brain cells (aka neurogenesis). New brain cells? Yes! Is not generally known, even by most doctors, that around 10,000 new brain cells are generated by the limbic system every night. Remember, the limbic system is what generates both emotions and memories.

You may have heard of mad cow disease? This is a condition where prions can cause shape mimicry in other proteins but happen to be resistant to the normal breakdown mechanisms. When you contract mad cow disease, you have been exposed to prions that rewrite the proteins in your brain and thereby cause havoc. But it was discovered in 2015 by Eric Kandel of Columbia University that these shape mimicking prions are also the naturally made proteins that are used in routine memory creation.

Just as we discussed shallow water drowning to understand how breathing is maintained, let us briefly explore what this naturally occurring experiment teaches us about sleep's function. When a person has a broken form of this shape mimicking prion, he or she can have a very rare sleep dysfunction called fatal familial insomnia (FFI). A single amino acid substitution (a broken protein) causes this devastating and rare condition that's been reported in only 100 people. These people are unable to go deeper than Stage 1 NREM (the first 10 feet of the scuba dive) and so they can't ever form K-complexes and sleep spindles to create memories. This results in insomnia, madness, and death. They never get a good night's sleep. The implication is that prions in and of themselves are not at all bad. They enable memory formation and efficient sleep. Only the ones resistant to breakdown (mad cow disease) or not functioning (FFI) are bad.

How do we know that declarative memory is prioritized during the earlier cycles of theta/delta wave sleep? In a beautifully designed experiment, University of Lübeck, in Germany, researchers found that subjects showed improved memorization performance when they were given an incidental rose odor while consciously memorizing only if it was reintroduced during the slow wave sleep portion of the night. No such improvement was achieved if the person received the rose smell before sleep, during REM sleep, or if he or she received only the rose smell during slow wave sleep but not with the original waking memorization.[10]

So, during sleep, how does our consciousness decide what will get stored in declarative memory and what is ignored and forgotten? And what does all this have to do with telomeres and aging? Since you will only ever have one "hard drive," your brain has to efficiently recycle the space like a computer hard drive does. This means we have to defragment it, erase sectors, and write new ones. It makes sense then that there is a basic hygienic procedure that exists when it comes to neuroplasticity that causes neural stem cells to copy and certain cells to selectively die to clear up space on your hard drive.

How does the emotional meta tagging that we described in the previous chapter work with sleep? Stuff that didn't feel important to your mind, body, and spirit won't be memorized with new spindles and K-complexes, nor will these experiences appear in the storytelling dreams of REM sleep. But stuff that was emotionally meta-tagged as important will. To illustrate, suppose you were out driving and came to a red light today. While stopped, you hear and feel the thrumming bass from a neighboring car. Chances are this experience won't be retained unless you have a strong emotional reaction to the song or glance over to see an interesting driver. Unless you have strong emotional meta tags, the memory will probably not be recorded. Emotions are the way that we sort through all the day's "noise" to get to what we interpret as valuable or not. The nature and strength of the emotion determines if and how memories will be used when we sleep.

Without the neuroplasticity of the early cycles of theta/delta wave sleep, you would struggle to make new memories and erase old ones—your memory would be jumbled and inefficient and you'd lack focus and make mistakes. Fatal familial insomnia is the extreme example of this, where defective prions result in the inability to sleep and form memory; that would be like trying to write without a pen or pencil. For the rest of us, sleep deprivation is like trying to write on the same sheet of paper that you've already completely filled with writing.

REM Sleep Is Where Active Learning Happens

Many animals might not need to create or weave complex stories and game theory models from their daytime experience. That nuanced ordered thinking comes from mirror neurons and the pesky need for playing nice with other unpredictable and dangerous humans. Most animals just need to remember who is the alpha and run on what we would call instinct. But a sneaky human might need to figure out how to get on the alpha's good side and then undermine him or her. That complex storytelling and software revision is the domain of REM sleep and procedural memory.

In the second half to two-thirds of the night's sleep cycles, the procedural memory is prioritized. Procedural memory is the assembly of information into a story, sequence, or skill. It is the learning of a *procedure* that is created during this active REM dreaming: like how to hit a baseball, read a poem, or be a friend to someone. The mind is engaged, the eyes move rapidly, and the autonomic nervous system is employed, which means your heart can race and you can generate emotional meta-tags during this dream phase. You are constructing stories or narratives out of thoughts, memories, and emotions. This is when beliefs of your subjective reality are constructed. In your nightly 3-D virtual reality, you are always teaching yourself something, so it is imperative that you meta-tag memory with abundance and gratitude rather than scarcity and recrimination. By using techniques like the C.A.R.E. method (see page 115), we can coax our demon thoughts to be more angelic. We see again that the TMTs cooperate to put you in an upward or downward spiral. Exorcise demons often and exercise what degree of self-compassion you can to tell better stories when you are dreaming.

Importantly, your body (except your eyes and diaphragm) is actively paralyzed so that you don't physically act out those vivid dreams. It is through the vivid virtual reality simulation of REM dreaming that we master skills, create meaning, and even form new declarative memories. That is why you can remember vivid dreams, although not often and not in great detail. The purpose of sleep after all is to use, or clear, old memories efficiently, not to recursively create more echoes of non-reality-based thinking.

Going back to our traffic light/loud music encounter: Let's say the stranger in the neighboring car makes an appearance in your procedural memory formation by way of a dream. What kind of dream will you have? Herein lies the importance of the concepts introduced in Chapter 5 on the mind. If you tend to filter your world with fear and scarcity, you'd probably have a nightmare; maybe you'd dream that the stranger scowls at you and assaults you in a fit of road rage. However, if you spend the majority of your mind's energy on flowing with gratitude and presence, possibly the dream you'll have will create a wonderful meeting with a kindred soul. How we "emotionally meta tag" daytime events can be modified by the C.A.R.E. technique of clearing, auditing, reframing, and enjoying. If we do a good job of creating abundant and grateful emotional meta tags, we can best leverage our dream life so that the procedural REM dream function can make us beliefs that best serve our goals of being the best versions of ourselves.

So during the later cycles of sleep, your consciousness works on your subconscious "issues" and manufactures meaning and narratives around the emotional turmoil, heartache, and triumphs of the waking life. If you aren't able to complete this vital task of sleep and dreaming, you won't be able to let go of your past, or to rewrite your history. It will be difficult to adjust to life's changes because you'll remain stuck in old stories about the world, others, and yourself. This leads to addictions, mood problems, and a poor quality of life.

If you are only getting 2 to 3 cycles of sleep (3 to 4.5 hours), you might not even accurately remember events. If you are getting 4 to 5 cycles (6 to 7.5 hours), you may remember the faces and some of the names but won't be able to subtly interpret them.

But if you are getting 6 cycles or so (more than 8.5 hours), then you might have the ability to remember people and events as complex, emotional, and nuanced parts of your reality. If you are a Silicon Valley tech CEO surrounded by sycophants, you might only need your own opinions, but most of us also must nurture the more evolved phases of spiritual dream life so that we can play nice with others. Remember the "theory of mind" from the last chapter? Well REM sleep allows us to put our theories about others into a simulated practice.

A final note: more is more when it comes to sleep. I do not believe you can oversleep, assuming your hypersomnia is not secondary to some undiagnosed other condition.

If you are the kind of person who has convinced herself she can't sleep more than five or six hours a night, then realize that naps can add up in terms of benefit; just think of countries that take siestas and how much fun they have. Historical records also indicate that there were times when many people slept in two phases, like six hours sleeping earlier in the evening, followed by some time up during the middle of the night, and then a few hours again asleep after that. Not everyone in these modern times has a lifestyle to accommodate multiphasic sleep habits, but some people swear by them and they are not necessarily incompatible with a stable 24-hour circadian rhythm.

THE OBSTACLES, CHALLENGES, AND SOLUTIONS TO GETTING GOOD SLEEP

The 5 A's: Anatomy, Anxiety, Ambien, Alcohol, and Alarm Clocks

Everyone has problems with sleep from time to time. Problems with quantity and quality arise for a myriad of reasons. Broadly speaking, our problems come from anatomy, anxiety, circadian problems, and substances that affect our level of arousal, like sleep medications, alcohol, and other drugs. Let's take a look at the A's that hurt our Z's first. Environmental tweaks to maximize a good sleep environment will be discussed later.

Anatomy: Obstructive sleep apnea (OSA) is the most common anatomical reason for disrupted sleep, affecting nearly 50 percent of middle-aged men in one study.[11] It was once thought that only obese people suffered from OSA, but in fact the collapse of the airway can occur with any body type, although excess weight is a contributing factor. The problem arises when you lose active muscle tone while unconscious; the airway closes, causing difficulty breathing, which can be heard as snoring. As a result, folks with obstructive sleep apnea stop breathing, their oxygen saturation drops, their brain stem knows they are asphyxiating, and it jars them awake, many times an hour. That doesn't sound very restful, does it? Well, it isn't. Studies show that people with OSA have shorter telomeres, racing heartbeats, cardiac stress, and even increased risks of heart attacks.

Happily, the problem of sleep apnea can be ameliorated with weight loss if you are obese, and by lying on your side with a pillow between your knees (regardless of your weight). To prevent rolling onto your back, you can even put tennis balls into your back pockets. If you tend to sleep on your back, you also help to keep the airway from easily collapsing two ways: (1) by sleeping with your torso propped up on pillows at a minimum of 30 degrees or (2) by placing a rolled up towel under your neck to slightly extend your head instead of the usual flexion (chin toward chest). If these anatomical fixes don't work, you can do what I have done since 1994 and sleep using something called a CPAP (continuous positive airway pressure) machine. These portable machines can blow a silent, gentle stream of air that is heated and humidified into your nostrils (or less comfortably into a nose-and-mouth-covering mask like a fighter pilot). Perhaps someday everyone will use a CPAP machine because they reduce the work of breathing while not damaging the system in any way. I view it like taking an escalator versus taking the stairs, but the medical profession, even in the absence of any significant risk of injury, would view routine use of CPAP by more people as a violation of some misguided code of ethics. So, unfortunately, you need a doctor's prescription to get one, and to get that prescription you'll need a sleep lab study with horrible results. I cannot recommend surgery for sleep apnea because of the low cure rate, scarring, pain, and changes in your voice that can occur.

Anxiety is a difficult and pervasive problem for many people. What are we so anxious about? Well, unfortunately, as we discussed in the last chapter, people can be overly goal-obsessed and possessed by "demons" of negative thinking. Those automatic voices tell us to worry about money, career, love, family, and the world at large. If your mind is burdened with anxiety-ridden, to-do-list-centered, or emotionally laden thinking, then your moments of brief wakefulness between sleep cycles (which are often primed by the content of your dreams) can make it hard to go back to sleep. What is the solution? Chapter 4's TMT Breathing Exercises and Chapter 5's TeloMirror Mind-Hacks to start with. Try this to see how one TMT influences and affects another: Breathe in with the thought, "I am," and breath out with the thought, "enough." Next, use the C.A.R.E. approach to create antidotes for the negative stories: clear, audit, reframe, and enjoy. Later, I'll give you a "top 10 gratitude" list that is a very helpful sleep tool as well.

Ambien (zolpidem): This commonly prescribed class of soporifics (sleep producing drugs) is one that should be avoided at all costs. Many of these drugs are cleverly named with *Z* at the beginning (as in getting your ZZZ's), but they are drugs as dangerous as any addict might abuse. They produce tolerance (needing more and more to get a fix), dependence (difficulty sleeping without them), and withdrawal when you don't take them. Not much better are the anxiolytic (antianxiety) drugs known as benzodiazepines (like Valium or Xanax) and barbiturates. These drugs, ironically prescribed to reduce anxiety, can cause not only addiction with harmful withdrawal symptoms, but a rebound anxiety effect after the drug wears off—causing more and more craving for said drug, and an inevitable downward spiral.[12]

What drugs are relatively safe to take for short-term difficulty sleeping? An over-the-counter antihistamine like Benadryl or Unisom is okay. If you are changing time zones, taking melatonin is helpful, along with getting sunlight to naturally increase its release from your pineal gland. Melatonin is the *zeitgeber* (time giver) and I don't recommend it for daily use; in Europe, it is actually a controlled substance, and some people report day-after drowsiness and fogginess.[13]

Alcohol is many people's drug of choice when it comes to winding down at the end of the day, but we must also be careful here because research actually shows that booze before bed can disrupt your sleep.[14] Plus, alcohol can cause sexual dysfunction and dehydration and produce a temporary inhibition of glutamine. Hours after you've had a drink, glutamine rebounds, causing an increased level of arousal in the middle of the night by suppressing the production of GABA, a relaxing neurotransmitter you need for sleep.

The **Alarm Clock** is the greatest thief of sleep, but to succeed in robbing you, your alarm clock (or alarm on your phone) requires an accomplice—you. It should go without saying that if you stay up late partying on the weekends, you are inviting circadian rhythm disruption. You can make up for fewer hours by sleeping in, but you cannot fight your internal, nearly 24-hour clock. It is important to go to sleep early enough so that you can get at least five cycles of sleep (at least seven and a half hours). There are now alarm clock apps for smartphones that claim to monitor your movements and infer how deeply you are sleeping. Being awoken in the middle of a deep dive into a sleep cycle is not a good thing. If you are healthy, your body's natural circadian rhythm will wake you in between cycles if you set that intention mentally. When you set your alarm, calculate for eight and a half hours, and set the tone for an extra 10 to 15 minutes past your planned time (so eight hours and 45 minutes total). And by tone, I mean, something gentle, not jarring. With this plan, your mind and body will have time to gently and naturally wake up, rather than being jolted back into consciousness by a loud buzzer. If you have a snooze button and the urge to use it, then you should. You may be mid-cycle and need the extra time to reach the conclusion of a 90-minute cycle. In this case, the old adage could be modified to state, "If you don't snooze, you'll lose."

TELOMERE SCIENCE AND SLEEP

There are many studies linking sleep dysfunction with telomere dysfunction. The common themes are what you might expect.

Less Sleep Is Associated with Shorter Telomeres

In 434 healthy older men, less than 5 hours of sleep versus greater than 7 hours was strongly associated with shorter telomere lengths. This association had a 96.5 percent chance of being non-random, but was not seen in the women studied.[15]

Both Quality and Quantity Matter

Another cohort study of 154 middle-aged people (ages 45 to 77 years) confirmed longer telomeres in people reporting at least 7 hours of nightly sleep. Interesting, they found a correlation between the subjective quality of sleep and telomere length as well.[16]

Snoring Shortens Telomeres

A large registry analysis of nearly 2,000 Finnish people showed that snoring and sleep apnea were associated with shorter telomeres after controlling for other variables.[17]

This finding was corroborated by this cohort study showing that after accounting for confounding variables of body mass index, smoking, and blood pressure, the association of obstructive sleep apnea with shorter telomeres was strong (confounding is the apparent relation of two things because of a third thing you are not considering). It showed a "p value" of 0.001, or just a 1 in 10,000 chance of being random in nature.[18]

Although we may like to believe that sleep dysfunction in terms of quality, quantity, and apnea directly impacts telomere biology, we must always consider a confounding and a holistic interpretation with regard to all the TeloMirror Tools. In other words, it is likely that a person who sleeps blissfully eight and a half hours isn't the kind of person who is angry, overweight, and doesn't exercise. If we can think, exercise, and eat well, then everything will conspire to heal stem cells and lengthen telomeres via the mysterious benefits of sleeping.

PUTTING YOUR SLEEP TELOMIRROR TOOL TO WORK

In keeping with a focus on mastery of one's emotions and beliefs, let me make specific recommendations for TMT sleep exercises that may help you improve your sleep and your telomeres.

1. Sleep with Gratitude

Every night, I like to host a "top 10 things I'm grateful for," countdown in my mind immediately before that long night's journey into day. It takes less than a minute, but I have found that it is one of the best and most powerful "hacks" out there. I usually do the top 10 list like this: Numbers 10 to 8 always include specific things that my ego found "challenging" that day. Numbers 7 to 5 will be material things for which I am grateful. Numbers 4 to

2 consist of people whom I cherish, and number 1 is reserved for something that I alone can do. Here is an example.

Note that we start with the things that we decided to be angry or frustrated about:

10. That person in the white pickup truck who aggressively passed me and flipped me off—I'm grateful he reminded me to keep my focus on the entire road and even those behind me.

9. The credit card company froze my card—I'm grateful that the company is watching out for fraud.

8. The flat tire—I'm grateful that tire lasted longer than I expected and that no one was hurt by the lack of tread leading to the blowout.

The middle three (life could be a LOT worse):

7. I am happy to have a safe and warm place to sleep every night.

6. I am grateful to be able to take an enriching vacation with my family.

5. I am happy to have an income when many people do not.

The near-the-top three (people whom I love):

4. I am grateful for the kind and sincere remark my coworker made.

3. I am grateful for the encouragement my parents still give me.

2. I am grateful for the love that my (son, spouse, pet) brings into my life.

Number one: self-care (or why I'm special):

1. I am grateful for my unique ability to make someone I cherish feel loved.

What is the point? I do this because I found that my patients taking telomerase activators usually had excessively blissful or excessively frightening dreams and it depended largely on their general views about life (back to mind-set). I realized we can definitely "spin" how we feel about things in those suggestive moments right before sleep, and that it makes a huge difference. Remember being tucked in by a parent? It felt nice, right? And recall the warning never go to sleep angry at your spouse? That is because a negative emotion will create a negative story and belief through the power of procedural memory formation.

You should choose wisely what seeds of thoughts, feelings, and beliefs you implant right before sleep because they will grow into whatever you sow while dreaming. Just as in waking life, thoughts become actions become beliefs. We don't see the world as it is but rather as we believe it to be. Plant better thoughts before sleep and you will grow better beliefs.

2. Waking with Purpose

The following can be done after a stretch or during morning meditation, but I actually prefer to do it as the first thought to greet the day. Granted, this is done after a night of sleep, but it is a great practice to get into each morning, and will help you sleep better each subsequent night. Try this:

Before opening your eyes, acknowledge that a new day has begun, then take a few conscious breaths and visualize your day. Surprisingly, to visualize your entire day takes moments, not minutes. You might see yourself meditating, showering, eating, going to work, interacting cheerfully with people and your tasks, doing your exercise, returning important messages, and then returning back to your bed later tonight. The visualization can be rapid and shorthand, like having just a feeling or a premonition of success. You may find that your subconscious will expand certain sections as needed to give specificity and guidance. The visualization may also benefit from general cues like "be open to serendipity or seeing old people in new and positive ways." Like any great athlete or performer will tell you, to perform at the highest levels of flow you need to believe you can; in order to believe, you need to visualize every aspect of how it will feel and look like to do the wonderful things you have planned for your day.

3. Check Your Basic Sleep Hygiene

Experts used to warn against exercise and eating before sleep, but in moderation, I don't see any problem as long as you don't have gastric reflux and aren't doing 200 burpies after downing nachos and ice cream. A hot shower or bath, massage, or sex before bedtime can be helpful. Essential oils, soothing music, and reading are also great. Maybe you like to meditate before sleeping, and that's fine; just remember that sleep is the best meditation. You have five senses: sight, sound, smell, taste, and touch. Assuming it is safe to do so, you would do well to shut them all down if you could to avoid distraction and allow your mind and body to recover and rebuild. But because we don't sleep in sensory deprivation floatation tanks, what steps can be taken?

- **Sights:** You should have window treatments that block all light. Most of us do not wake with the sun, after all. If you have light contamination in your sleeping space, especially if you work night shifts, be aware that even your skin can sense light. Use a comfortable eye mask if needed. There should be little exposure to blue light from screens because it helps reset the circadian rhythm. Some devices allow you to filter out the blue light, which can be helpful. "Winding down" with three hours of social media or television is squandered time you could be using to enjoy the blissful repair and restoration of sleep.

- **Sounds:** I often sleep to a nice playlist of soothing music in the background. You can also download apps that will create noise in various colors as well as a plethora of natural, musical, and meditative sounds that are soothing. An even better alternative for most people is to sleep with ear plugs. Because I sleep with a CPAP machine and even the faint sound of air moving can be distracting during the brief awakenings between sleep cycles, I often like to have one or two ear plugs in place. If you are sleeping next to a person who snores or makes a lot of distracting noise, consider discussing CPAP or sleeping elsewhere, and definitely try those earplugs. Your mind can subtract most sonic distractions, but because it has better things to do, why overload your system with distractions that are irregularly irregular? If you do use a smartphone, please don't forget to shut down the electromagnetic output by going into nontransmitting or "airplane" mode.

- **Smells:** Hopefully, there aren't any odd smells in your sleep environment. Try to have clean sheets on your bed, and eschew plug-in chemical smell makers. Use of pleasant essential oils or light incense or candles is okay, if you extinguish them before sleep. Many people find frankincense, myrrh, and lavender relaxing. You might want to get those pets out of the bed, to say nothing of the babies (even with their fantastic baby smell).

- **Touch:** I believe everyone should consider sleeping without clothes, or with the loosest and lightest ones possible. In many climates, a choice of breathable sheets and lighter comforters is seasonally appropriate. I cannot stress enough the importance of temperature maintenance in your sleep. I prefer to sleep at a balmy 76 to 78 degrees Fahrenheit, and if the room is cooler or warmer than this, when I have a middle-of-the-night awakening, some action may be called for to change the temperature, which is an invitation to sleep disruption. Because your core temperature drops in the later half of sleeping (around 4 A.M.), you can invite problems if you don't have appropriate bedding and good ambient temperature control.

- **Feel (or Sleep Positioning):** Finally, although it isn't well appreciated, we have three curvatures in our spine and our thighs come out of our hips at an angle. If you sleep on your back, you should have pillows under your knees to take pressure off your low back. A thin pillow or even a small rolled up towel is best for under your neck because neck flexion caused by typical pillow use encourages airway obstruction and neck stress. If you sleep on your side, you should have a pillow between your knees to keep pressure off your low back as well (thighs will be parallel) and you can hug a fluffy pillow to support your arms and shoulders.

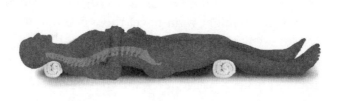

- **Taste:** Because of mouth breathing and failure to swallow saliva actively, the normal cleansing of the mouth doesn't occur efficiently while sleeping, leading to bacterial overgrowth and "morning breath." If you wish, you can keep a bit of water to drink next to your bed or even use mouth cleansing strips or spray between sleep cycles to keep your mouth cleaner and kissable. These small measures can help stave off needless fighting of low-level infections in your mouth, thereby preserving your telomeres as well.

CONCLUSION

Sleep is one of the most crucial things you can do to stay young, healthy, and, yes, beautiful. There is a reason they call it "beauty rest." Your body is repairing, your mind and spirit are healing and learning, and you get to drop all the pretenses of ego and the struggles with demons that constitute our haphazard and messy waking lives. If you had to choose one from all of the TMTs to focus on, getting the best sleep possible would likely be the most important one and the most neglected one as well.

Think of sleep as the mental defragmentation and spiritual shaking of the Etch A Sketch. It is the chance to reframe the bad, visualize the good, and commune with the rest of the conscious universe in the theta brain wave streams of unconscious knowing.

Sleep is like playing music, making love, or freestyle rapping. Everyone can do it. Not everyone can do it well. But there are steps you can take to learn and ways to increase your chances of success. Good luck.

In the next chapter, we will move from restoration to active destruction. We will discuss everyone's (including the late Jack LaLanne) least favorite thing to do: exercise. But it is through the act of destroying our bodies that we can rebuild them into stronger and healthier homes for our mind and spirit.

Chapter 7

Your Exercise

The heart is made of muscle. Muscles
grow stronger with use and can't be broken.

For many, exercise is pleasurable; it releases natural opiate and cannabinoid chemicals in the brain and body. As a TMT, it leverages and improves the other tools by providing us the opportunity to breathe deeply, exorcise demons, and enjoy more restful sleep, and it makes us look good and feel good about ourselves.

Ostensibly, the purpose of exercise is to stress, stretch, and actually damage the muscles, ligaments, tendons, bones, and arteries at a low level so that they will be compelled to rebuild themselves into stronger versions. Given the destructive and sometimes uncomfortable nature of this endeavor, would people still exercise if they didn't have to and could just pop a pill to achieve the same benefits? After all, millions of people already enhance their workouts with anabolic hormones like testosterone derivatives and human growth hormone.[1]

And why did Jack LaLanne, America's consummate evangelist for exercise and fitness, make the following rather disparaging remarks about exercise?

"It's a pain in the glutes, but you gotta do it . . .
I hate working out. Hate it. But I like the results."[2]

WHAT IF "WORKING OUT" OUT WAS CALLED "PLAYING OUT"?

Why can walking to work seem like a burden, whereas walking up a mountain or along the beach doesn't? There are so many wonderful ways to play: sports, exploring a new city, dancing, riding waves, snowboarding, skiing, and biking. Your body is working, but we don't often consider these activities "working out" do we? Our minds create a false dichotomy, which I believe the cranky Jack LaLanne was alluding to, something along the lines of: there is stuff I HAVE to do because it is "good for me," and stuff I WANT to do because it's fun.

Why are some movements more fun than others? Maybe because fun connects us with people, has a freshness or pleasurable quality about it, or is a challenge that puts us into a high performance "flow" state, as discussed in Chapter 5. Just think about how grateful to exercise you'd be if you were paralyzed or if you lived in a prison cell like a factory farm animal. As with mental fitness, you can begin to shift attitudes about exercise by tapping into a more mindful and grateful outlook for all you are able to do. Whenever you move, you can choose to be mindful, which will increase your mastery and calm by focusing on balance, breathing, presence, and pleasure of being alive and in motion.

In previous chapters, I called into question the notion that our reality is based solely on the material world. When it comes to exercise, we must also conclude that we are more than mere mechanical machines. Think about it: the more "work" we give any of our other machines, the faster they break down. Why is the opposite true with a body? Because unlike machines that import replacement parts, our organs produce new and better replacement parts from stem cells after the older ones are wiped out by exercise. Creative destruction is how exercise renews us and how the system operates. When you injure muscle fibers by lifting weights or doing sit-ups, your body adapts by making new muscles if the existing muscles were not adequate to easily complete the task.

WHAT IS THE PURPOSE OF EXERCISE?

We are adapting creatures and so we have to use and even overuse our bodies to be in shape. Just as we will discuss in the next chapter on diet and weight, the body is designed to maintain homeostasis (maintaining the status quo), so it is often hard to build up to a new level. But there is an upside to the tendency toward homeostasis: it is equally hard to lose physical conditioning from lying around for a few lazy days.

A moralist would say you have exactly the body you deserve based on the work you have put into it. However, it's more accurate to say that you adapt to the body you require for the actions you perform. Of course, the process of "aging," which you now understand to be the degradation of telomeres and stem cells throughout your body, does make it more difficult to maintain fitness. But if you had to rank them, it would be hard to put exercise far below any other TMTs in potential benefit. Perhaps sleep, reframing with gratitude, conscious breathing, and laughter would challenge for the top spot, but it is undeniable that exercise generally makes people look and feel younger. How does it do that? Well, exercise releases hormones for anabolic growth (like testosterone and human growth hormone), relieves anxiety and depression, makes you breathe efficiently, and activates both opioid and endocannabinoid pathways for bliss. Simply put, all your cylinders fire better when you rev those engines.

So, must we consider movement as work? I'll grant you that running, biking, or climbing to nowhere on a machine in the gym, all the while having your mind rendered flaccid by watching TV, seems suboptimal to me. Let us consider exercise to be an essential part of living as much as sleep, food, and breathing. Be grateful you can move in ways that not everyone can and feel good that physical activity helps your telomeres, stem cells, and whole body to remain in top condition.

THE BASIC MECHANICS OF EXERCISE—HOW IT WORKS

Our bodies are truly amazing. Let's spend a moment to review how we command and control movement, how the cardio-pulmonary system (your heart and lungs, the plumbing and ventilation) works to keep you pumping along, and finally how the structures of your body function, with an emphasis on muscles, joints, and bones.

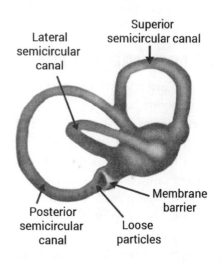

Command and Control

Control of movement is achieved with several neurological systems in your brain and your body. First, we have real-time monitoring via our sensory systems; this includes proprioception (the awareness of posture and the locations of body parts in space), balance (largely regulated by the cerebellum [a mini-brain at the rear of the big brain], and 3-D spatial awareness via visual imaging and three semicircular canals residing in your inner ears that are aligned on three axes: X, Y, and Z.

To move, your brain sends outgoing signals that we know as the voluntary motor system. Your brain commands you to "lift your arm" and the arm complies. But don't be fooled—there are countless flavors of that command, such as "lift your arm to hit a tennis ball," "lift to grab the last slice of pizza," or "lift to shake a friend's hand." These are complex scripts that we "learn" via procedural memory and that comprise many subroutines of ritualized and coordinated movement. But these procedures aren't just static commands; they involve real time sensory input to adjust on the fly: "a safe toss in the wind for the second serve," "grab the pizza from your brother who has already made a move," or "change handshake to a fist bump when you realize your friend just sneezed into his hand."

In addition to the countless scripts of movement, we take for granted that there are also postural muscles of the trunk and even muscles in the lower extremities that can run on automatic without conscious thought. Even though we don't realize it, try standing on one foot and you will understand that even balancing at rest is a very active and complex process. Ironically, the procedure of "standing still," involves many subroutines of subconscious monitoring, engaging of muscles, and fidgeting.

The Plumbing and Ventilation

Some of our discussion about breathing in relation to exercise will be familiar to you from Chapter 4. In order for efficient movement to occur, there are metabolic costs you must pay. The following processes are always occurring, but the demands of exercise intensify this process. You use your lungs to inhale fresh oxygenated blood that is delivered to the left side of your heart. The left side of the heart, along with the pulsating arteries, then propels the red oxygenated blood throughout your body so you can move and your body can work (or play). Also, circulation means that blood is also carried to the skin for evaporative cooling (aka sweating). Much of the oxygen is used in the tissues and the hot, less red, and deoxygenated blood is now full of acid-producing CO_2 (from the cellular metabolism) and returns via one-way veins to the right side

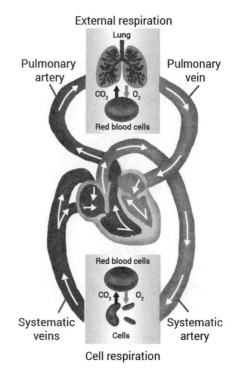

External respiration

Lung

Pulmonary artery

Pulmonary vein

CO_2 O_2

Red blood cells

Red blood cells

CO_2 O_2

Systematic veins

Cells

Systematic artery

Cell respiration

of your heart. From there, the right side of your heart pumps the blood back into the lungs for CO_2 release, heat dissipation, and a fresh supply of oxygen to bind to the hemoglobin of the red blood cells.

Your cardiopulmonary function constantly adjusts by balancing between the excitatory **sympathetic** (fight-or-flight) system, and the relaxing **parasympathetic** system (see Chapter 5 for a review). When you exercise and exert more energy, your sympathetic system tells your heart and arteries to pump stronger and faster and the airways dilate to allow better ventilation. The parasympathetic does the opposite.

Your body constantly regulates your blood pressure from one beat to the next in real time. There are pressure sensors in your neck arteries and aorta that transmit information to the brain stem to adjust the relative influence of the sympathetic signaling, making the heart pump harder and faster, and the parasympathetic, causing the heart and arteries to pump more gently and slowly when the pressure is excessive.

If the blood volume is too low, a different method is used to increase it. There are sensors in your heart and neck arteries that increase salt retention by getting the hypothalamus (the hormonal control center of the brain) to release a hormone known as antidiuretic hormone (ADH). The ADH signal tells the kidneys to retain salt and water, which increases blood volume.

So, what if we are getting the proper blood pressure and volume to where we need it, but we still have low oxygen levels from cellular respiration and inadequate inhalation? (Remember Chapter 4's TMT of breathing? It's all related.) Think of running on a treadmill while holding your breath; even the idea of it might make you feel dizzy. Well, oxygen sensors in your neck arteries and the large artery leaving the left heart known as the aorta are constantly monitoring your oxygen levels. With low blood oxygen levels, a signal goes to the brainstem causing us to breathe faster and deeper.

If we exercise too much without blowing off adequate CO_2, we become acidic from the by-products of cellular metabolism and the increased carbonic acid from the CO_2. Just as low oxygen in the blood is detected by arteries, any drop in the pH is immediately detected by the brain stem itself, which will increase breathing rate and depth, even if you are in a coma or brain dead as explained in Chapter 4.

Your Body Mechanics—the Machine, as Such

The way your body moves is a complex and beautiful system. Let's take a look.

There are 206 bones in a human body that serve as the scaffolding that enables movement. Bones are also the storage sites for the body's calcium, but after our 20s, our bones grow weaker. After menopause or "andropause" (a controversial term for the decline of male sex hormones in advanced age), the loss of bone density and strength accelerates. Of course, lack of load bearing from prolonged bed rest, even among healthy young people, also allows for loss of bone density and strength. If you don't use it, you lose it.

That said, both hormones and active load bearing from exercise help to maintain bone strength. Interestingly, there appears to be a direct correlation with telomere shortening and pathological bone thinning, as shown by a study of telomere lengths in bone.[3] These researchers had actually proven my stem cell theory in osteoporosis, but because they assumed leukocytes (or white blood cells) were some universal measure of aging, they didn't even recognize the importance of their findings and reported their study as a negative result. As my epigraph in Chapter 5 stated: "Seeing isn't believing. It works the other way around." They couldn't see the truth of there being only one disease with many faces. They had proven telomere shortening in the bone caused osteoporosis despite having normal white blood cell telomere lengths, and they were unable to see it because they lacked the belief system to understand it.[4]

Most of your 206 bones are connected with other bones in connections known as **joints.** Joints come in many shapes and functional designs and they can have ligaments, fibrous and fluid filled capsules, cushioning cartilage, and stabilizing muscles attached by tendons. You need bones connected to joints and muscles in order to exercise.

Joints tend to have limited blood supplies, making repair slow and often problematic. The **cartilage** in joints makes up the semi-solid, spongy spacers and placeholders that allow them to slide and rotate with high efficiency and low friction, instead of having rough bone rub against rough bone. If cartilage tears, like the common meniscal tears of the knee, even a hairline tear can cause pain and be slow or unlikely to heal due to the poor vascularization of these areas. It is important to avoid injury to joints by observing proper mechanics and by listening to your body when it is in pain.

Ligaments are connective tissue connecting bone to bone whereas **tendons** connect muscle to bone. A common ligament tear from exercise or too much physical stress is the anterior collateral ligament or the medial collateral ligament of the faithful but challenged joint we call the human knee.

A little stress from exercise improves the strength

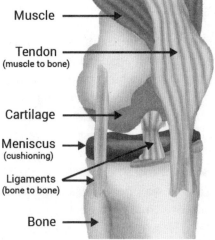

Muscle

Tendon
(muscle to bone)

Cartilage

Meniscus
(cushioning)

Ligaments
(bone to bone)

Bone

and resilience of your bones, cartilage, ligaments, joints, and muscles. Muscles are particularly good at becoming stronger with destructive behavior (i.e., the tearing down of muscle fibers through exercise) as long as you don't go too far and rip your tendons off your bones.

It is the damage and inflammation of sore muscles from strength training that prompts the niche muscle stem cells that are known as satellite cells to work to produce more muscle cells.

Muscle proliferation in the heart and arteries is also stimulated by exercise. Some research suggests a direct link between low oxygen levels triggered by aerobic exercise and increased telomerase activity.[5]

Once again, the paradox of fitness is that your bones, skeletal muscles, pumping heart, and pulsing arteries adapt and get stronger mainly by being challenged with the stress introduced by exercise. When you challenge your body to adapt to a higher level of activity you are adapting to a higher level of homeostasis. Thankfully, an analogy with car maintenance fails us when it comes to exercise, which is quite interesting. Unlike car parts that all degrade from stress, friction, oxidation, and electromagnetic waves, your body will actually grow stronger with a modest level of abuse as long as you give it time to recover and repair. What accounts for this critical difference? Younger and better replacement parts for our bodies are constantly available from our mesenchymal stem cells (remember, these are undifferentiated stem cells that can become muscle, ligaments, and bone when needed) as long as you don't push too hard. Figuring out just the right amount of stress is our next topic.

OPTIMAL FUNCTIONING FOR EXERCISE

Optimal functioning when it comes to exercise varies from person to person, and it basically boils down to finding out what sort of exercise works for you. That means identifying what is enjoyable, safe, but also challenging. The other part of optimal functioning with exercise, is that when you do discover what you love to do, do it as often as you can. But choose wisely. You can't have it all. If you decide that you love power lifting, you won't be able to also follow a plan for becoming a great marathon runner. If competitive tennis is where your bliss is found, then you might have to give up on bulking up for that maximum dead lift competition.

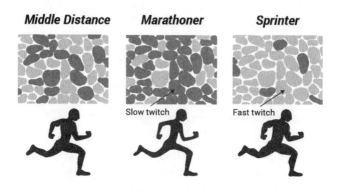

Don't like to exercise at all? If you sit at a desk for 12 hours a day, your body is adapting to that activity with strong postural muscles and probably some forward hunching of your shoulders and neck. This adaptation will cause poor breathing, neck and back pain, and that can't be good for your telomeres, right? If you don't like to exercise, find ways to do what you need to do with an increased level of physicality. Bike to work. Take the stairs. Get a standing desk. There are ways of creating habits that increase your need to exert yourself.

Not everyone agrees with Jack LaLanne, you know. Some people enjoy and even crave exercise. Those folks may be somewhat addicted to exercised-induced endorphins, which are natural opiates released when exercising. Opiates are molecules that produce pain relief and euphoria. So exercise can be considered a socially approved form of drug addiction! Why do people want euphoria? Whether they know it or not, maybe this "runner's high" is another way to exorcise demons of consciousness while also exercising their bodies. There is a catharsis that can happen during exercise that helps you to transcend automatic and obsessive thoughts that can seem to be constantly running your life.

So, to find your own personal optimal functioning with regard to exercise, start by asking yourself what you want your ultimate goal to be when it comes to fitness. Do you want to look good in a bathing suit? Maybe thrice-weekly weight training and a low glycemic diet is the way to go in that case. Do you want to compete in triathlons? You'll need to do a lot of aerobic training and maintain a low body fat percentage to avoid joint wear and tear. Want to use exercise to help you live longer? Then maintaining a moderate body fat percentage with a balanced approach to strength, flexibility, and cardio may be the best.

Whatever your physical performance needs or aspirations may be, your body will adapt as long as you have decent stem cells to replace damaged ones. As the years pass, you may be losing performance because you are replacing your cells with just marginal stem cells that have aged along with you. In the future, as we will discuss in the final chapter, you may have the option of freezing high quality, personal, and even gene-restored stem cells. In that more optimal scenario, when you break down a muscle, tendon, or joint, your replacement cells will be closer to factory new than the versions that you've been carrying around for all these years.

When it comes to optimal exercise functioning in regard to keeping your telomeres young, we should observe several principles. Finding what you like, as I already mentioned, is part of the equation. Some personality types prefer discipline, repetition, and routine. Others seek fun and variety. Once you identify what you like, there are three major components to consider when choosing exercises:

- First, it is good to have some cardiovascular challenge.

- Second, we seek muscle overloading with "muscle confusion," (or mixing it up to benefit from adaptation to the new), and allowing for some days of recovery.

- Finally, you should encourage flexibility without inducing injury.

Other exercise considerations that can improve your life and longevity include exercising in ways that allow you to spend time with people and pets you love, to meet new people and socialize, to release stress and focus the mind, and to get some sunlight to make vitamin D.

Cardiovascular Training or "Cardio"—Getting Your Juices Flowing

The category of "cardio" means exercise for the heart and lungs. The idea is to get the heart pumping a lot of blood to predominately slow-twitch muscles, which are responsible for performing low intensity, repetitive motions over relatively long periods of time. Typical cardio activities might include brisk walking, running, biking, and swimming. Cardio is an activity that gets you winded, gets your heart racing, and makes you sweat. Your cardiopulmonary efficiency and joint stability generally dictate how intensely and how long you can go. Like everything, this efficiency tends to decline after your 20s and that decline accelerates with non-use.

At the center of the cardiovascular system is, of course, the heart. The heart is an amazing organ and can become very strong as long as the valves and electrical circuitry remain healthy. It is one of the few organs that rarely get cancer, and as long as the arteries remain clear, your heart can grow quite strong from intense exercise even at an advanced age. Unfortunately, the arteries tend to harden, and to lose elasticity and pumping efficiency in advanced age, so even with a world-class heart, a decline in performance can be anticipated.

What is the best form of cardio as we get older? It is probably swimming because of the low levels of stress on joints like knees and hips, and the wonderful connection to water. Did you know that the word *spa* comes from the Latin for "health from water" (*sanus per aquam*)?

Pumping Iron: The Quest for a Chiseled Body

Resistance training comes in endless varieties: simple calisthenics using the body's own weight as resistance (such as push-ups, sit-ups, and jumping jacks), lifting weights like medicine balls, kettle bells, dumbbells, free weights, machine resistance, plyometrics (jump training), and interval training (alternating bursts of activities with rest periods). These routines can cross over with cardio in many forms although the common theme is that they seek to engage more of the fast-twitch, burst muscles in an effort to increase strength, mass, and definition. If you never push your muscles beyond what is comfortable, you will simply maintain what you have. Our bodies only adapt to change, and if there isn't a change in our routines, we won't adapt to a new normal. Just like if you memorize the same 1,000 words, your vocabulary won't increase, will it?

WARNING: It is imperative that you learn the biomechanically proper ways to do any exercises to limit the chance of injuries from repetitive stress and improper loading. Most experts recommend weight training no more than three times a week unless you are rotating body areas (like taking "leg days"). They believe that the breakdown of muscles requires at last two days of recovery in order to be of maximum benefit. It is during rest times that the hormones are surging and the stem cells are copying your bigger and stronger muscles and other tissues into existence. In my experience this recovery time can be decreased and healing efficiency increased when patients take telomerase activators or adaptogens, as we will discuss in Chapter 9.

Yoga—The Ideal Telomere Maintenance?

For those seeking flexibility and serenity, yoga is a great choice. It is a form of moving meditation that is based on conscious breathing while moving through relatively static poses. Yoga, when properly practiced and instructed, can be modified to nearly any level of fitness, strength, and flexibility. Many studies show that yoga is superior to many other forms of back pain treatment.[6]

In the West, yoga continues to evolve to include entirely new postures; to introduce weights and cardio; to incorporate acrobatics and partners; and even to bring in elements such as meditation, chanting, aromas, and healing sounds called "gong baths."

As a nearly daily practitioner of heated yoga group classes since 2011, I can attest to the increased energy, calm, and preserved flexibility and strength that the practice fosters. I know that being among positive, breathing, and conscious people moving to music is a way of achieving balance and flow in my own life. I have never left a class, no matter how hard the workout or what chaos pervades my life, without more energy and calm, so I am probably just as much of a "junkie" for endocannabinoids as runners are for opioids.

In yoga class, you can see a wide range of ages and body types that thrive and gradually transform with it. Good yoga teachers are like artists, because it is not generally a lucrative career, but rather a calling; they all have stories of personal transformation of the body and the way of living. Interestingly, the word *yoga* in Sanskrit means to join, as in joining oxen with a *yoke*. It is a way of creating integrated balance and flow, so in a practical sense, it is like having many TMTs working at once—exorcising demons, cultivating presence, mindful breathing, challenging exercise, and enhancing compassion and self-care that radiates outward.

In the final analysis, all movement constitutes exercise. Try salsa dancing on a Friday, swimming solitary laps when it's hot, riding stationary bikes with urban professionals when it's raining, or hiking the mountains with your dog on a Sunday morning . . . it's all wonderful.

So remember there is no sitting on the bench and you absolutely get a trophy for participation when it comes to the work/play/sport of movement as an adult. But as we get chronologically older, we must take care to be safe while pushing the edge of what we have comfortably achieved. By pushing for greater feats of strength, endurance, and skill you will be able to keep your body young, your heart and lungs efficient, and your hormones healthy and in a growth and regeneration mode rather than decay.

COMMON PROBLEMS WITH EXERCISE AND LONGEVITY

One serious problem with trying to live forever by exercising is the tragically ironic phenomenon of sudden death. In this scenario, a middle aged, sedentary man decides to get in shape, but the plan backfires when he drops dead from a massive heart attack. It happens—so the lesson is to give your body a chance to gradually adapt to a higher level of challenge or risk injury or worse.

Always get evaluated for palpitations, persistent shortness of breath, excessive fatigue, tingling and numbness, nausea, and persistent pain. If you encounter chest pressure and shortness of breath from a flight of stairs, get a stress test. That will mean putting you on a treadmill or stationary bike while monitoring your heart's electrical patterns and your vital signs to make sure that you don't have unstable angina (inadequate blood perfusion of the heart muscle by clogged or inefficient arteries).

Another common problem is injury. Challenge yourself but always pay attention to your body because pain should never be considered "weakness leaving the body," as some weekend warriors like to say. Pain is inflammation from injury and is a warning to stop doing what you are doing. You should know the difference between muscle fatigue and pain. If you decide to ignore and push through pain, you will be prone to injuries to Achilles tendons, wrists, rotator cuffs, and knees; those kinds of common injuries will keep you from benefiting from exercise while you recover and defeat the purpose, don't you agree? Only highly paid professional athletes routinely play through pain and they often suffer late season and career-ending consequences for it.

Inadequate recovery time can also be a problem. Strength training involving muscle destruction and, without recovery, more exercise is just more destruction. Repetitive stress of ligaments, tendons, joints, and bones follows the same principles. We need time for adequate healing to benefit from exercise, and as we discussed in the previous chapter, sleep is the prime time for growth hormone and cell replication to take place.

Finally, boredom and lack of discipline are not uncommon problems. If we are honest, lack of time isn't really the root problem. If everyone did a few dozen push-ups and sit-ups with good technique and some stretching, that might take all of five minutes a day. With just that modicum of exercise, we could all look great in a swimsuit assuming we didn't eat too much. But alas, we over-complicate, ritualize, procrastinate, and create imaginary barriers to fitness.

TELOMERE SCIENCE AND EXERCISE

There are many studies that look at telomeres and exercise. Unfortunately, the majority of them look at just the white blood cells because they are easy to measure—but these studies wrongly assume that white blood cells can reflect aging in general. Actually, every organ has its own stem cells and there are studies demonstrating that white blood cell lengths don't correlate well with telomere lengths in other organs. Think of cars in Chicago versus San Francisco and you would expect different rates of damage from road salt and parking brake usage. A coal miner has shorter telomeres in his lungs and an alcoholic has shorter telomeres in his liver.

As with most studies, we can only guess at causal mechanisms. What we can assume is that people who exercise engage many positive "upward spiral" lifestyle habits that have holistically positive effects. People who exercise have decided that life is worth the effort, which is hopeful. Regular exercisers possess discipline, life organization, and drive; they enjoy better hormone function, improved self-image and appearance, possibly better social interaction and integration; and exercisers experience some healthy cellular destruction and regeneration.

All that said, lets look at just a few of the better studies out there and see what general conclusions we can draw about the relationship between exercise and leukocyte telomere lengths (as a presumed, but flawed proxy for biological age).

Mix 37 Studies in a Blender and You Get a Meta-Analysis

A meta-analysis is a scientific smoothie of sorts. You take disparate studies and attempt to combine them with some statistical slight of hand into one really big study. I don't believe such a technique is very sound, but my opinion is in the minority. One 2015 meta-analysis attempted to combine 37 studies of exercise and telomere length. Twenty of the included articles did not find any statistically significant association between exercise and leukocyte telomere length (which could be due to a lack of statistical power or sufficient numbers of subjects), whereas 15 did show a positive association. Two papers showed an inverted *U* and one of them is the last paper we discuss in this section.[7]

The Greater the Variety, the Better the Results

One of the best studies was a large cohort study published in the journal *Medicine and Science in Sports and Exercise* in 2015. The researchers analyzed the data of 6,503 people, ages 20 to 84, in the National Health and Nutrition Examination Survey, and found that self-reporting revealed that all types of exercise, after adjusting for other factors such as age, were associated with longer telomeres. The types of movements were recorded as moderate intensity, vigorous-intensity, walking/cycling for transportation, and muscle-strengthening. People who engaged in at least two of the four types of movement-based behaviors had significantly longer telomeres.[8]

Sorry, There Is No "Glory Days" Effect

A study of 815 Berliners showed that practicing sports for at least 10 years had a very positive impact on telomere length. Of note, the researchers point out that exercise had to be in effect since age 42, suggesting that with the onset of middle age, the practice and effects of exercise become more powerful and critical.[9]

In this study, a history of being an athlete in one's early adulthood did not confer a benefit; this lack of benefit from the remote past was corroborated by a 2015 study of elite former Finnish athletes.[10]

Nice Legs—Nice Telomeres

An interesting 2015 study published in *Medicine and Science in Sports and Exercise*, found that the ability to walk long distances and having powerful leg strength were correlated with increased telomere length, when compared with no walking.[11]

Breath Is Life

In contrast to the performance and physical conditioning results of a 2010 study published in *Mechanisms of Aging and Development* suggesting that the oxygen carrying capacity of the subject, or the VO_2 max, was the only variable correlated with telomere length. This could be confounding with a global effect of aging and breathing, but probably also suggests that in addition to immunity, the ability to breathe is associated with being vital.

The Smoking Gun for Telomeres and Overdoing It

If you don't believe that you can overdo exercise, consider the Fatigued Athlete Myopathic Syndrome (FAMS). A 2003 study by Collins et al. in *Medicine and Science in Sports and Exercise* showed that muscle biopsies from these athletes were significantly shorter and that this disease was directly correlated with critically shortened telomeres, suggesting that the muscle stem cells were being required to copy so frequently that they didn't have time to regrow the length. Unlike most studies looking at white blood cells, this study examined the actual cell type in which telomere shortening is producing cellular dysfunction and disease.[12]

Moderation Is Best

As mentioned in the study of 37 studies, at least two studies concluded there is a "U-shaped" curve between exercise and benefit. Too little exercise is bad, but too much, as in the case of FAMS is also potentially bad. Ludlow et al., in their 2008 study in *Medicine and Science in Sports and Exercise*, showed moderation was best.

Telomere length was best in those who didn't overdo it or neglect their exercise.

GETTING THE MOST OUT OF YOUR TELOMIRROR EXERCISE TOOL

The best exercise is that which makes you feel alive and connected and encourages you to adapt to being efficient, strong, and flexible. The dividends of playful and purposeful movements will include a happier endocannabinoid system, younger stem cells with longer telomeres, better sleep, better self-image, improved love life, enhanced mood, and better mental and work performance.

The research indicates that exercise is most critical after age 42. You should do exercise in moderation that includes strength and resistance training as well as aerobic challenge. A good goal would be to make sure you are strengthening your legs and using your breathing capacity. Whatever your passions, hobbies, pet situation, and commuting look like, give yourself adequate recovery time and don't exercise a joint or muscle that is still in pain. Here are some ways to incorporate more exercise into your telomere preserving routine.

1. Pick a Social Activity—or Not

Some people prefer to exercise alone. Other folks crave variety and social interaction. If you are in the latter group, there is always a group exercise class out there for you, such as dance, calisthenics, or yoga.

2. Make It a Mindful Routine

I personally love daily hot yoga because I breathe deeply, sweat, and maintain flexibility and some strength and balance. Some of the other mindful movements are tai chi and qi gong. If you are doing cardio exercises, varying the intensity with interspersed rest periods, known as interval training, adds focus and improves the efficiency of what you're doing.

3. Create a Habit

You can set up a cue, routine, and reward for your exercising. For example, set your gym bag by the door to remind you or set a smart phone alert. After completion of your workout, you can get a smoothie or coffee to positively condition yourself.

CONCLUSION

As we continue to build upon breathing, mind-set, sleep, and exercise, I hope you are starting to grasp that everything we are discussing has been shown to help telomeres and that all these behaviors and beliefs work together. After all, we are integrated holistic organisms, seeking balance and flow. If you only desire to be healthy, your choices, breathing, dreams, movements, and eating will conspire to make *you* the placebo effect, as Dr. Joe Dispenza tells us in his book *You Are the Placebo*. And the placebo effect is very, very real; only what we believe about ourselves can be observed and manifested.

We close with another quote from the late health guru, Jack LaLanne: "Exercise is king. Nutrition is queen. Put them together and you've got a kingdom." But always take care that the king and queen are cooperating. You can exercise with too low a body fat and suffer consequences, which may have contributed to avid running guru Jim Fixx's death. You can be consuming excessive calories and be overweight; this makes exercise dangerous with an increased risk of coronary artery disease, joint injury, and accidents. You can have an amazing physique but if your cutaneous body fat percentage is too high, no one will see the definition in your muscles, if that matters to you.

There are a lot of notions about nutrition out there, many of which are based in truth and which most avid fitness fanatics usually love to share with you. This is a good segue to our next chapter on the fifth TeloMirror Tool: Your Diet. The good news about nutrition is the same as the bad news: you probably overthink something that is inherently pleasurable and beneficial. There are general guidelines you can follow to improve your food choices so I hope that you approach the ones in the next chapter with an open mind, and that you welcome the good news: food is good for you and an invitation to enjoy your life more blissfully.

Chapter 8

Your Diet

"We must eat fruits and vegetables to live."
— No Eskimo, ever

If we really are what we eat, why don't we eat people to remain human? I think this chapter may be the most challenging to read, because we harbor so many incorrect beliefs about eating. We feel responsibility for what we put in our bodies because we believe the people selling the notion that nutrition is critically important for good health. What if I told you that the human body can adapt to nearly any kind of diet and that your body's degradation comes not from what you eat, but from the loss of telomere length? The latter isn't necessarily informed by the former in exactly the way you'd think, and the truth is that humans can survive on just about any sort of diet. Of course, to survive is not the same as to thrive, so it will be up to you to find what foods improve your health. As with all TMTs, our goal is to first understand, then grant ourselves the agency to find our own wisdom.

Most people's core belief can be summed up by Jack Lalanne's statement "Exercise is king. Nutrition is queen."[1] Certainly there are some foods that are better for you than others, but I believe the composition of your diet, assuming you aren't poisoning yourself in ways we will discuss later in this chapter, may be the least important aspect of staying young when compared with breathing, mind-set, sleep, and exercise. Having said that, we will draw upon the current state of telomere science to suggest food and dietary habits that may be associated with better health.

But first, it's important for you to learn some basics about nutrition, digestion, metabolism, and biochemistry. Don't worry, we will keep it simple and no one is going to quiz you. This is adult education meant to enrich, not stymie you.

Much of what we were taught about diet is flawed. People are now starting to appreciate that the food industry demonized fat and promoted sugar and wheat. We now understand that you don't get fat from eating fat any more than you get high cholesterol from eating cholesterol or get smarter from eating brains. To your metabolism, fat is just a more concentrated form of calories and there is the same amount of energy in 1,000 calories of animal fat as in 1,000 calories of vegetable fat, or 1,000 calories of bread, which is full of supposedly fattening carbohydrates.

THE PURPOSE OF EATING

We eat so that we can supply our body with glucose, a simple sugar. Remember when we learned about cellular respiration in Chapter 4? We encountered the coin-operated Laundromat machine analogy and learned that all our energy-requiring reactions are powered by "quarters" of ATP. Well, the only bills the change machine of metabolism accepts are $1 bills of glucose. Protein, carbs, and fat are like $2, $5, and $10 bills that need to be exchanged for singles to make ATP. What I mean to say is that your body doesn't use protein, carbs, and fat directly as a power source—instead it converts all of them into one-dollar bills of glucose that are used by the cellular change machine to make quarters.

ATP, or adenosine triphosphate, is related to the DNA molecule called adenosine. Throughout our bodies, chemical reactions use

ATP to power movement, synthesis, and countless other actions. A single molecule of glucose, via processes called glycolysis, the Krebs Cycle, and oxidative phosphorylation, makes up to 38 ATP. Most of those come from oxidative phosphorylation inside the mitochondria, which are the thousands of symbiotic former bacteria that provide energy from within each one of your cells. I say "former" because it is believed that mitochondria got incorporated into our ancestors' cells 1.5 billion years ago. Interestingly there are only five grams of ATP in your body but each individual molecule is recycled about 600 times daily, amounting to the consumption and reconstitution of your entire body weight worth of ATP daily. That could be compared to doing your entire neighborhood's laundry with only a single roll of quarters.

Your body has the ability to convert nearly anything you eat into nearly anything you need, so what you eat is not as important as you might imagine. Our bodies are like airport currency exchange kiosks in that they can "eat" or receive intravenous glucose, and then synthesize glycogen (a short-term storage form of glucose kept in muscles and the liver), proteins, and fats. Conversely, we can just consume fat and by means of gluconeogenesis (the formation of glucose) we can get all the glucose we need even without ingesting it in a process known as lipolysis (or fat breakdown).

Having said all of the above, some foods and diets are safer, more nutritious, and easier on our bodies than others. Hopefully, someday we may all consume food with fewer pesticides, hormones, preservatives, radiation, additives, and DNA fragments called plasmids, prions (like those that cause mad cow disease), bacteria (like salmonella from eggs), and viruses (like hepatitis A in seafood). Perhaps the food of the future will be engineered to be pure, easily digested, delicious, and safe. Just like anything, including water, can be harmful if taken in excess, natural food contains a myriad of molecules that can get into your system and which are chemically processed, or "detoxified" if you will, by the liver in a process described below.

Pure Protein Diet: The Exception to the "It's All Good" Airport Kiosk Rule

As we discussed shallow-water drowning to better understand breathing and fatal familial insomnia to understand sleeping, let us now turn to a rare form of malnutrition that occurs to understand eating: rabbit starvation. This was described when carnivorous humans tried to subsist on overly lean meat and historically occurred among people in Arctic climates who didn't have access to marine sources of meat that are rich in fat.

The protein overload that can occur from eating a diet of meat that is overly lean (like rabbits) or eating animals from late in the winter season (which are low in stored glycogen and fat) is toxic. Fat gives us 9 kilocalories per gram (kcal/gm), so is an efficient mode of energy intake and storage. Not that you care, but *calorie* is just a scientific term for the amount of energy required to raise a kilogram of water one degree Celsius at sea level pressure.

Consider this example: If a person needs 2,000 calories per day and is eating only meat without fat or carbs, this would equal 500 grams of protein (like carbohydrates, protein provides 4 calories per gram weight). Digestion of this amount of pure meat, mostly composed of protein and the amino acids that come with it, produces more ammonium than your kidneys can excrete daily. Symptoms of such a rabbit starvation diet would include diarrhea, fatigue, low blood pressure, headache, and, not surprisingly, a craving for fat. Interestingly, a diet of pure carbohydrates or fat doesn't produce biochemical problems like rabbit starvation from protein overload. Eating pure protein is the exception that proves the rule that we can survive on any kind of diet.

HOW DIGESTION WORKS

From Food to Nutrients: Mechanical and Chemical Digestion

It seems inefficient when you think about it, but eating and digestion serves to mechanically and chemically break down and then absorb foods into the smallest, simplest components, only to be reassembled into the same complex molecules for our internal use. This is because food contains such a wide range of potentially toxic agents that we can't just let it in safely, like an intravenous hamburger. In the next few pages I hope to explain everything you need to understand about the process. We're going to start with the food you put in your mouth, and follow it through all the phases of the digestive process. By the end of this section, you'll have a clear and concise understanding of your entire gastrointestinal (GI) tract (from your mouth to your anus).

The Mouth: It all begins in the mouth. You use your teeth, tongue, and entire mouth to mechanically break up food into smaller particles, which allows for more efficient digestion. Saliva contains three enzymes that aid in the chemical breakdown of sugars (amylase), proteins (protease), and fats (lipase).

From Mouth to Stomach: The esophagus is a nonrigid muscular tube that uses undulating waves to push food down toward the stomach.

The Stomach: Your acidic stomach has a pH of 2 owing to the production of hydrochloric acid that dissolves and disinfects the food you eat. This caustic chamber uses tight muscular sphincters to regulate the intake and outflow of food, which keeps acid from gurgling upstream (causing heartburn), or downstream (causing a duodenal ulcer). If the mucous protection fails, it can lead to a peptic or stomach ulcer.

The Liver: Another important part of digestion, your liver uses green, soapy **amphiphilic** (both water- and fat-soluble) molecules stored in the gallbladder, known as bile salts or bile acids. These bile salts surround nutritional fats and fat-soluble vitamins (A, D, E, and K) and transport them to the bloodstream. Your liver receives all the blood from the intestines like a giant swimming pool filter, and detoxifies substances before they enter your bloodstream. It does this in two phases: First, by a chemical breakdown called oxidation, reduction, and hydrolysis; and second, by adding side groups to the surface of toxins (creating conjugated toxins) required for wastes to be excreted in the urine or feces. These conjugated toxins and **bilirubin** (a common breakdown product of red blood cells' hemoglobin) are disposed of via bile into your GI tract. If bilirubin accumulates in a malfunctioning liver, the skin and eyes show yellowing known as jaundice. Proper circulation of bile between the intestines and liver is essential to rid the body of toxic waste and to enable absorption of fat-soluble nutrients and vitamins.

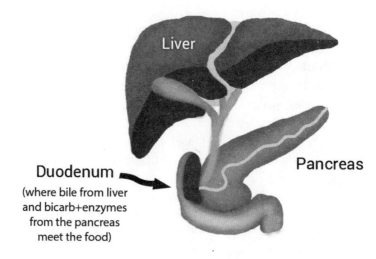

Liver

Pancreas

Duodenum

(where bile from liver
and bicarb+enzymes
from the pancreas
meet the food)

The Duodenum: The first part of the small intestine, the duodenum, is connected to the exit of the stomach. It is a C-shaped "carwash" about nine inches in length, which lies above the pancreas. The duodenum has a single spigot called the **ampulla of Vater** that sprays food with bile from the liver and gallbladder, bicarbonate from the pancreas (corrects the acidic pH imparted by the stomach's hydrochloric acid), and digestive enzymes from the pancreas (the same enzymes that are released in saliva). This process changes the acidic pH of 2 to a basic pH of 9, which is the pH required for digestion to continue.

So fats are absorbed with soapy bubbles of bile. Simple sugars are absorbed from the gut into intestinal cells by active transportation through specific channels, one single sugar molecule at a time. Proteins are also transported in a similar way, although the "necklace" of proteins must be chemical digested into component "beads" or amino acids. Amino acids are not absorbable if they remain longer than four amino acids. There are 20 amino acids and 11 of them can be manufactured; so the other nine **"essential amino acids"** are like vitamins insofar as they must be ingested. Although it may seem inefficient to disassemble, absorb, and then reassemble the proteins, it serves to protect us. This is why you should be wary when people suggest that specific proteins like growth factors in bone broth can have significant health benefits when taken orally. They can be absorbed by vesicles at a very low level but in general, most large proteins do not survive chemical disintegration.

The Pancreas: Your pancreas acts like a thermostat for your important blood sugar level (aka blood glucose level) by producing two opposing hormones known as **insulin** and **glucagon**. When blood sugar is too high, the pancreas releases insulin that quickly lowers blood glucose by forcing it into cells to be converted into and then stored as fat. When blood sugar is too low, the pancreas produces glucagon, which raises the blood glucose by signaling the cells to make those "$1 bills" from coins or to break larger bills of fat and complex carbs called glycogen into singles.

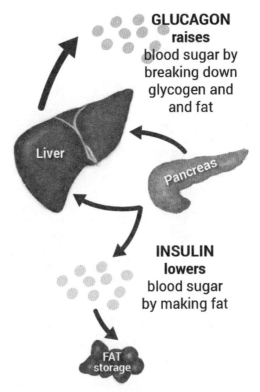

GLUCAGON raises blood sugar by breaking down glycogen and and fat

Liver

Pancreas

INSULIN lowers blood sugar by making fat

FAT storage

If glucose is like bite-sized segments of licorice, **glycogen** is made up of long ropes of glucose like licorice whips. Glycogen is depleted after several hours of fasting (or sooner if you are exercising). It is this depletion of reserve glycogen that wakes up newborn babies, who can't store glycogen before four months. That's why they wake up instantly "hangry" so frequently. Loss of glycogen is also what makes long distance athletes hit "the wall." After glycogen is depleted, you maintain blood sugar mainly by eating fresh carbs or breaking down fat. That is the reason why **ketogenic** diets and other high-protein eating plans, such as the Atkins diet, cause you to melt fat. Eating pure fat makes you shed fat because contrary to what intuition would tell us, there is a thing called biochemistry.

Many single glucose molecules
assemble to form glycogen...

...a polymer of glucose in chains

...just like single licorice bites
could be assembled into long ropes

The Small Intestine: Once the food leaves the duodenum, it enters the first half of the small intestines. The first eight feet of this narrow diameter intestine is known as the **jejunum**, and it looks like a coiled and undulating tube, lined on the inside with microscopic shag carpet, or villi. Your villi, like the tendrils of a sea anemone, are where the simple building blocks of amino acids (deconstructed from proteins) and sugars (deconstructed from polysaccharides) are actively transported across the intestinal wall.

The next 10 feet of small intestine, known as the **ileum**, looks similar to the jejunum from the outside and has similar villi on the inside, but this part of the GI tract is specialized for absorption of vitamin B12 and the soapy bubbles called micelles, which are packages of fatty acids surrounded by bile salts and phospholipids (the molecules that make up cell walls).

The Large Intestines: The last five feet of the GI tract, called the **colon**, or large intestine (for its wider diameter), ends at the anus and serves mainly to concentrate stool into hard clay by reabsorbing precious water. If your intestines need to get rid of something toxic or irritating and it is too late to vomit it back up because it is already beyond the ileocecal valve, you'll experience diarrhea (water-laden stool), which is your body's way of rapidly flushing toxins out.

In contrast to the large intestine that is full of bacteria, after most of the work of your digestion is done, the contents of your small intestine are relatively clean unless you have something called SIBO, or small intestinal bacterial overgrowth. We do host bacteria in the large intestines to make vitamin K and further process bilirubin into molecules that lend the yellow color to urine and the brown color to feces. Relatively clean small intestines and dirty large intestines are why your colon is equipped with a one-way ileocecal valve so the downstream stinky, bacterial-infested poop doesn't flow backward, like a toilet backing up.

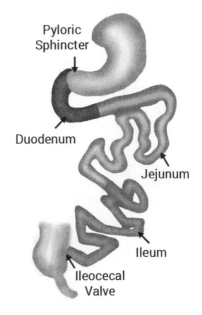

Pyloric Sphincter

Duodenum

Jejunum

Ileum

Ileocecal Valve

To review: eating and digestion serve to mechanically and chemically break down and then absorb foods into component smaller molecules for absorption. Toxins, bacteria, and indigestible substances are excreted as hard clay known as stool.

After reading the preceding few pages, you already know all you will ever need to know about digestion. Now, let's move on to higher-order questions of how we regulate the process.

HOW HUNGER WORKS

Before the wonderful central nervous system evolved, evolutionary theory suggests that our predecessors were little more than tubes specialized for feeding. It follows that there was an enteric nervous system, or "gut brain," before there was a spinal cord and central nervous system. The enteric nervous system has learned to interact with the central nervous system however, especially through the autonomic nervous system that we discussed earlier. Low blood sugar is a primary way in which the autonomic nervous system is triggered to induce hunger.

The main signal of hunger is a good example of hormonal communication between the gut brain and the normal brain. When your stomach is empty, its cells produce the hunger hormone known as **ghrelin** that tells the "mission control" room of the brain, the hypothalamus, that you should eat something. When the stomach is stretched by a meal, the ghrelin production is suppressed. Knowing this, we can "hack" our hunger response and potential overeating by keeping the stomach stretched out with more water (still zero calories, by the way) during meals. We can also decrease ghrelin by eating something every few hours to reduce the time the stomach is empty.

Although immediate hunger is signaled by ghrelin, the long-term modulation of hunger is controlled by two hormones produced by fat cells known as leptin and adiponectin, which were first discovered in 1994 and 1995 respectively.

When we eat a meal, we release cholecystokinin (the word means "gets the gallbladder moving"), which serves to decrease appetite, delay stomach emptying, reduce acid, release pancreatic enzymes, and signal the liver and gallbladder to dump into the carwash.

Good health means optimum function and balance of existing systems. We should be careful what we wish for when it comes to inventing appetite suppressants. It is possible that creating chemical blockers of the signaling done by ghrelin, leptin, and adiponectin may help control obesity in the future, but why risk tweaking a working system using what many bring forth unwanted and dangerous consequences? One comical example is Orlistat, which prevents fats from being absorbed; the unavoidable consequence of trying to fool Mother Nature is anal leakage of oily stool. If we have properly functioning stem cells that are appropriately dying off and being replaced when damaged, then we will enjoy better energy utilization and homeostasis of weight.

It seems obvious that normal appetite is not the root problem leading to obesity. Is shivering a problem of being cold or hypersomnia the cause of depression? What if obesity is not primarily a consequence of the types and amounts of food that we consume, but rather a result of the aging of cells?

In 2007, after just three months of taking a telomerase activator, I lost 15 pounds without diet or exercise, and I have maintained this happy new weight despite eating like a kid and not exercising. From that experience, I concluded that some massive dysfunctional stem cell extinction event must have occurred in my visceral fat that needed three months of non-stem cell replication (the Hayflick limit of replicative senescence) to manifest. The replacement of aged fat stem cells with younger ones (and therefore longer telomeres, or slowed shortening of telomeres) led to a shift in the food digestion and storage economy referred to as metabolism.

There is a phenomenon called metabolic syndrome, or Syndrome X, that is characterized by central obesity, insulin resistance, inflammation, and serum high lipids such as cholesterol. I believe that stem cell aging is the cause of this condition, which is just an extreme example of what happens to all of us to some degree as we grow older. Getting fatter may simply be a result of stem cell aging, caused by telomere shortening and mutation across all cell types, but particularly in cells of the liver, pancreas, and visceral fat (belly fat).

There is only one disease with many faces.

Do you remember that *I Love Lucy* episode where Ethel and Lucy were working on a chocolate assembly line? Well, think of your aging cells as line workers that take up cholesterol and other nutrients it passes by. When they are damaged and less active, they don't use the building blocks of cholesterol at such a high rate anymore, and instead of small bags of fat (high-density lipoprotein or HDL), you get big bags of fat (low-density lipoprotein or LDL). The entire story of "bad cholesterol" may be erroneous because it may represent an association formed by confounding. Both low rates of cholesterol usage and adverse clinical outcomes are associated with cellular aging due to telomere erosion. The fact is that the majority of people don't have certain rare mutations in their lipoproteins that confer higher rates of atherosclerotic complications.

Although we can and should resist, my theory of aging suggests that obesity is as inevitable as the aging of stem cells in other organs leading to dementia, high blood pressure, and diabetes. Without adequate telomerase activity and telomere preservation, our fat stem cells accumulate genetic damage. Without efficient destruction and replacement of those damaged stem cells, each TMT cylinder function degrades: troubles breathing, difficulty staying positive, sleep apnea, reduced exercise, and eating habits that bolster obesity.

If we prevent our stem cells from becoming damaged from telomere shortening, their daughter cells will be more metabolically active, like efficient, young, and fast-working chocolate factory assembly-line workers, and we will get less fat accumulation, insulin resistance, and high lipids. Think about how hard it was to gain weight as a teenager, and yet how easy it is as the years pass by. What if the pizza-proof body of a teenager is merely the result of relatively undamaged stem cells from having preserved telomeres, and a therefore more efficient metabolism? Homeostasis is merely metabolic inertia. A teenager finds it hard to gain calories despite eating 5,000 calories; an old person finds it hard to lose weight despite eating 1,000 calories. The key is not calories in but rather the metabolic needs of the system and its capacity to maintain homeostasis given the relative health or degradation of its cells genetic and epigenetic programming.

On a more global and holistic scale, we should also examine addictive behavior patterns, mood problems, and the types of food that we choose to ingest. This is a good segue to a topic of major importance—the glycemic index, which is a critical concept to understand when it comes to controlling our risk for obesity and diabetes.

What Is a Glycemic Index and How Does It Relate to Ketogenic Diets?

When you refrain from eating carbs and then consume your several hours' worth of available stored glycogen, your body goes into a process known as ketosis, which is the breakdown of fats to make glucose triggered by the pancreatic glucagon mentioned above. Daily marbled rib eye with butter equals rapid fat loss. Daily marbled rib eye with a soft drink equals obesity. If you can endure not having any sugar in your diet, your body will be coerced into breaking those "hundos" of stored fat to come up with singles of glucose and the quarters of ATP.

Next to the magic of the photo-editing programs, the Atkins or any ketogenic diet is the best friend of cover models and actors everywhere because in no other way can you melt away fat so quickly. It may take weeks, but there is no way to avoid looking ripped if you melt fat of the surface of muscles by avoiding carbs.

Remember when I suggested that 1,000 calories is 1,000 calories, regardless of source? Well that wasn't entirely true once we understand the concept of a glycemic index—which is the efficiency with which a food raises your blood glucose.

Unless you are planning a hunger strike or survival competition, 1,000 calories of maltose from beer IS a lot worse for you than 1,000 calories from lard because of its higher glycemic index.

Maltose in beer is made up of two glucose molecules, so it is like getting a double shot of glucose. Glucose is ready-to-use energy and the high glucose leads to insulin release and fat storage. Now you understand where the term *beer belly* comes from. In contrast, lard needs to be broken down, absorbed, and converted into glucose before being reassembled into lard, which doesn't occur efficiently in the absence of a high glucose level and resultant high insulin levels.

Evolutionarily, this was a very good thing because high glucose meals were few and far between when we were hunter-gatherers. But with today's sugary drinks and starchy food, it is a recipe for the obesity of modern life. Glucose has a glycemic index (aka GI) of 100 percent. This means that 100 percent of the glucose you absorb is reflected immediately in your measurable blood glucose. In contrast, fructose, the sugar in fruits, raises your blood sugar only about 20 percent. For your reference, sucrose, or refined table sugar and high fructose corn syrup (commonly added to snacks and soft drinks) raise your blood sugar with about 70 percent efficiency.

Monosaccharides, or single sugars, such as glucose and fructose can also come in pairs, such as table sugar or sucrose (which is glucose plus fructose) or lactose (galactose plus glucose).

To avoid fat storage, the worse thing you can do is to have high glycemic foods in binges, like eating a handful of candy. All things being equal, it might be better to spread out that same handful of candy over six hours. That way you won't get a massive increase in blood sugar that will induce insulin release and glucose conversion and storage as fat. It's not just the "area under the caloric curve" but the peak that you produce over any given period of time that matters.

To avoid storing fat in our modern world, it is better to eat lower glycemic foods like nuts, meats free of antibiotics and hormones, and organically grown fruits and vegetables. It is preferable to have a variety of delicious, minimally processed foods. All the other trace minerals and essential amino acids, essential fatty acids, and vitamins will be extracted from your diet assuming you have a good variety.

IMPACT OF FOODS ON BLOOD SUGAR

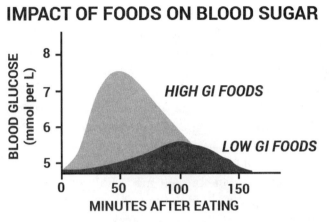

What is bad food variety? The foods from the center of the supermarket, engineered to remain unspoiled for months to years, have chemical preservatives and those chemicals are not great for you. On the other hand, the outside aisles of the supermarket have perils from pesticides if not organically grown, weird coatings like alar on apples, and sometimes high bacterial counts in the case of perishable items like eggs, milk, and yogurt.

Since we can't generate ATP using photosynthesis, as plants do, we must ingest energy by eating. Interestingly, a caloric intake far below or exceeding our ideal requirement doesn't produce changes in our body composition because our body seeks to maintain homeostasis. If you need 2,000 calories but only take in 1,000 daily, the weight loss will be slow (unless you are in a ketosis state) and if you take 3,000 calories instead of 2,000 daily, the weight gain will also be gradual as well. The ability to maintain homeostasis on the macro scale is correlated with youth so the older you get, the harder it is to stay the same weight. That's because your gene expression, cell integrity and cooperation, and organ function are all changing. Youth is wasted on the young! It is easier to stay young when you are young and easier to grow old when you are old and you are becoming less like yourself in every way.

As mentioned earlier, it turns out that as omnivores, we are metabolic currency conversion kiosks. We can thrive on pure meat diets, as did the Inuit or Eskimo people, or pure vegetable diets, as do many health-conscious Westerners and nearly half a billion Indians. The good news is that there's a wide range of choices in regard to healthy diets, as long as you don't deprive yourself of certain nutrients, such as vitamin B12, which can be low in a vegetarian diet.

Evolutionarily, there aren't really good and bad foods, so the adage of "you are what you eat" is not accurate. If that were the case, we would all have to eat humans, and in most cultures, that is morally the worst food! Sadly, humans dichotomize most things as good or bad and therefore our food choices are either good or bad. What if we just understood our choices and weren't so hard on ourselves? It makes me sad to hear people say, "I went to the gym, so I can be bad," when they eat something delicious but forbidden. There is so much self-judging without true understanding. It is as though people want to be slaves to guilt.

In order to eat for better energy and healthful outcomes, perhaps we just need to be more mindful; perhaps the automatic thinking we discussed in Chapter 5 is at fault? Maybe a habit of pizza, pastries, coffee, and so on holds too much power over us if we define them as morally good or bad?

What if, instead of counting calories, you just thought about becoming a conscious eater, enjoying beloved food in smaller portions, with plenty of water to expand your stomach? What if you consciously ate when hungry instead of by the clock and never felt guilt about leaving some on the plate? What if you kept healthy snacks on hand to eat every two to three hours and drank lots of water between? This would keep your stomach stretched out and would suppress ghrelin production, making you feel less hungry. What your parents called "spoiling your appetite" (snacking) actually curtails the negative impact of scheduled binge meals with their sudden and taxing dumps of food to ingest, digest, detoxify, metabolize, and store. Think of how tired you get after a big meal, which is fine if you are planning a siesta and catching up on your REM sleep, but not so good if you have things you need to do efficiently and on a schedule.

We probably evolved as hunter-gatherers, constantly eating. In modern times, our parents spent a large amount of time and effort on scheduled, labor-intensive meals with social significance. But as adults, we usually have choices and should leave the guilt of spoiling our appetites or hurting the cook's feelings by the wayside if we are to become more mindful about eating.

If you must adhere to the false dichotomy of good versus bad foods, the literature regarding diet and telomere health points in several directions that will appeal to you. In general, the research as explained below eschews sugars and saturated fats and extols vegetables, fruits, seaweed, and omega-3 fish oils. The more inflammation and oxidation producing foods of sugars and grains are shunned in favor of the anti-inflammatory and antioxidant foods particularly found in the Mediterranean diet.

COMMON GASTROINTESTINAL MISTAKES

One big problem we face is that many convenience foods that are affordable, available, and taste good tend to produce inflammation, have highly caloric fat, and also contain glycemic sugars, which induce insulin release and the storage of excess glucose as fat.

I believe that unconscious food behaviors may be the biggest nutritional problem: people grow accustomed to eating the same foods, from the same sources, at the same times, in the same configurations. As you will learn in Chapters 10 and 11, keeping a daily self-inventory is a great way to collect objective data so that you can be more mindful about your life, including what you eat, how often, in what quantity, and why (hungry, bored, or stressed). A food being delicious is a great reason to eat it, and it is a pleasure not to be denied oneself, but emotional and addictive eating can also lead to overeating and obesity. Strategies coming up in the next section will show you how to be a conscious, mindful, and therefore healthy eater.

Swimming Cramps: Not an Urban Myth

Don't exercise after a big meal. Remember being warned by your parents not to eat and then swim? Well, if you jump into a cold pool, you will need to pump blood to your muscles and skin and rob it from the intestines. While a small meal will wait patiently for the GI tract to come back on line, a big lunch will not sit well, resulting in those "cramps" that you get. Conversely, increased blood flow to the GI tract is also the reason for feeling cold after a big meal; the blood isn't going to your skin, but rather to your digestive core.

Skip Colonics

Somewhere along the way, people got the notion that the colon was like an ancient clay pipe, lined with old debris. They decided that rinsing the colon would be a good way to eliminate "toxins." Releasing toxins is something we constantly and naturally do in every cell with antioxidants, with every heartbeat delivering blood to our liver and kidneys, with every breath we exhale, and with bladder emptying and bowel movement. Colonics are done by using a tube inserted into your rectum, which is then used to flush large amounts of water, and sometimes herbs or coffee through the colon. Not only are these procedures entirely unnecessary, they can be harmful. Having seen the inside of colons during colonoscopy, I can attest that the notion that there are caked-on deposits is a load of you-know-what. Colonics also increase your risk of dehydration and infection, can cause bowel perforations, and can be harmful to your heart and kidneys. Bottom line: Skip colonics!

Food Pyramids Are Marketing Hype: Ignore Them

Historically, agribusiness influenced government recommendations via professional lobbyists because they had a lot of wheat, corn, and milk to sell to consumers. It was only as recently as 2011 when the U.S. Dietary Association ditched the decades-old food pyramid with which we were inculcated. That pyramid suggested we take the majority of the diet, or the base of the pyramid, from grains, which are filled with glycemic carbohydrates and gluten, which some people are sensitive to. Even our American "superfood" of milk was business propaganda; cow's milk is not a great choice for humans, because many are intolerant of its lactose, it contains antibiotics and casein, and it has been associated with higher rates of cancer, osteoporosis, and acne, according to some research.

The new USDA pyramid, or plate, now emphasizes more plant-based eating over processed grains, which is good. Unfortunately, the science is still flawed and the recommendations are rather arbitrary. Perhaps the mission of this government agency is too broad and that they can't serve as an agribusiness advocate, consumer health advocate, and impartial authority? It is not their fault however. There is no such thing as an ideal diet any more than there could be a list of the best 10 movies to watch or 10 songs to have on every playlist.

Why did people even care what the USDA thought? Well, most of us want to believe in authority (it's easier), and many of us are motivated to act in ways that are "good," versus "bad." The truth is that notwithstanding food sensitivities and allergies, most people do well with a variety of foods. How can you make a USDA recommendation to the effect of "everything is fine in moderation"?

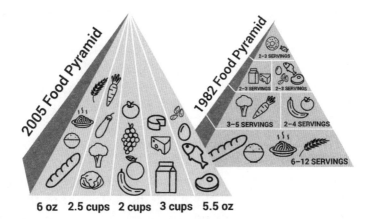

The Morality of Consumption: Why So Guilty?

Speaking of moderation, perhaps the sanctimony around exploiting other species can be tempered. Factory farming of fish, poultry, and cattle raises serious safety and food quality problems. Since we can now technologically replace meat from animal slaughter with mass-produced beef, poultry, and pork from stem cells grown in a lab without sacrificing living animals, is that also a form of existential cruelty from nonexistence? The questions are not as simple as they might seem. If you could ask cows before they are incarnated whether they preferred to be born and slaughtered or not born at all, what would the reply be?

Many people are vegan because they don't want to exploit animals. I once heard a comedian say, "I'm vegetarian not because I love animals but because I hate plants." I don't know if plants personalize their destruction, but they might have a form of consciousness. I once had dinner with a couple that practiced Jainism, a religion based on nonviolence. They questioned the way in which the lobster I was eating had been prepared (by boiling alive). So thought I would counter by asking about plant consciousness and using soap to kill bacteria. They vanquished me by informing me that their priests shower with water only and eat only fruits that fall to the ground naturally.

It is difficult to eat without exploiting other species at present. Technology may change that soon, but until it does, we should find ways to create sustainable, natural, and blissful conditions for plants and animals to exist before they are harvested.

So if there is no such thing as an optimal diet, what should you eat? The good news, and the answer is that you can enjoy anything that is safe, affordable, delicious, and has a good variety. Don't get caught up in magical beliefs about alkaline diets, Paleo eating, tracking macro- and micro-minerals, or looking for the "life force" in foods. As we will discuss in the next chapter on supplements, your body is designed to extract what it needs in terms of minerals, calories, vitamins and essential fatty acids, and amino acids. Just be grateful that unlike breathing, thinking, sleeping, and exercise, nature has deemed that digestion is too complicated and important to be left to your voluntary control. Your system automatically takes care of all the currency conversion for you and you won't be the worse for it. You think Paleo is the way to go? Just consider that the average life expectancy in the Paleolithic era was 30-something.

TELOMERE SCIENCE AND NUTRITION

When we discuss nutrition and health, it becomes nearly impossible to control for confounding variables. A *confounding variable* is a third, unexamined variable that explains the statistical association between two factors that you found. For example, when people are vegetarian, they might enjoy healthier telomeres. But if vegetarianism is also associated with healthier weight, meditation, yoga, mindfulness, and other positive and telomere-positive behaviors, then we are at the mercy of statistical design to discern the direct and true relationship between vegetarianism and telomeres.

Life is complex—as are our bodies. We function best when happy from the molecular to the spiritual level. Having stated this disclaimer, scientists do have a favorite theory about nutrition and telomere health and it is branded as the anti-inflammatory Mediterranean diet, which is rich in fruits, vegetables, whole grains, nuts, legumes, olive and canola oil, herbs, and favors fish and poultry over red meats.

All Kinds of Studies Agree: The Mediterranean Diet Is Best

A large cross-sectional cohort study: eating Mediterranean-style diets appears to increase telomere length, say researchers from the Harvard School of Public Health who studied over 4,600 nurses. The study, published in the *British Medical Journal*, found that following a Mediterranean diet was associated with longer telomeres.[2]

A nonrandomized prospective trial: The hypothesis of an anti-inflammatory Mediterranean diet was verified by a nice

5-year prospective study, which is a rarity in clinical science. In this Spanish study, 520 people at 0 and 5 yrs with high cardiac risk were tested at baseline and then they were allowed to eat what they wanted. Those with the lower inflammatory foods had the slowest rate of telomere shortening.[3]

A cross-sectional study of elderly patients: In 217 elderly Italians, the intake of a Mediterranean diet, after controlling for age, gender, and smoking habit, was independently associated with LTL (p=0.024) and telomerase activity levels (p=0.006).[4]

A multifaceted cohort study looking at inflammation and oxidation: In a Chinese study of 556 patients with prediabetes, there was already an association with poor glycemic control and shorter telomeres. They failed to show a correlation between dietary fat and carbohydrates and LTL, but there was a proven negative association with sugary drinks. As the above studies suggest, this study also found a positive association with legumes, nuts, fish, and seaweeds and longer telomeres.

Comment: What made this study even more interesting is that they attempted to isolate the effects of certain food types on inflammation and oxidation. Total calories, higher fat and carb diets, cereals, and meats were associated with increased inflammation.[5]

Processed Meats Cause Inflammation and Telomere Shortening

In a study published in *The American Journal of Clinical Nutrition*, collaborating researchers from universities in Texas, Vermont, Seattle, Minnesota, and Norway found that processed meats such as hot dogs, bacon, and many common lunch meats appear to be particularly harmful to your cells. The study's investigators analyzed the eating habits of 840 men and women, ages 45 to 84, and found that telomere shortening was seen even if people only ate processed meat once a week, compared with those who avoided it altogether. For each additional serving of processed meat, telomeres shortened further.[6]

No Surprise Here: Obesity Is Associated with Shorter Telomeres

Obtaining or maintaining a healthy weight preserves the health of your telomeres, according to researchers from the University of Medicine and Dentistry and St. Thomas Hospital in London. The study investigators, who recruited more than 1,100 women, ages 18 to 76, measured their telomeres, and recorded their weight status, found that lean women had longer telomeres, while heavier women had much shorter ones. The researchers also noted a direct relationship between leptin (a hormone associated with hunger and obesity) and shorter telomeres.

Comment: The problem here is how much of weight is associated with other powerful confounding variables such as the other TeloMirror Tools: impaired breathing, sleep dysfunction, depression and anxiety, lack of mindfulness, dearth of exercise, and so on.[7]

Does Changing Eating Habits Help Our Telomeres?

As discussed in Chapter 7, when researchers at UCSF looked at obese women and attempted to intervene with teaching mindful eating, body awareness, meditation, and yoga, two very interesting things happened. First, even the women who didn't receive the treatment benefited, indicating that knowing they were part of a study made them somehow receive a powerful placebo effect. Secondly, both treated and untreated participants experienced higher telomerase activity and improvements in stress, cortisol, dietary restraint, and food choices.

Comment: Although the researchers would have obviously preferred their intervention to be very different among the treated and untreated groups, the bigger picture is even more empowering to us all. The lesson is that just making the decision to improve something (e.g., joining a study, in this case) triggers improvement even in the absence of the learned tricks and practices that were supposed to make such a profound difference. We are the placebo, indeed![8]

HOW TO GET THE MOST FROM YOUR TMT DIET

The theme of relative nonchalance about nutrition in this chapter might seem as ridiculous as the comedy of Woody Allen in his classic movie *Sleeper*. Woody's character woke up in the future after being cryogenically frozen with his old 20th-century beliefs about health and nutrition. In his 20th-century life, he owned a wheat-germ-selling health-food store in Greenwich Village. Amusingly, when he starts to become anxious from the stress of waking up in an unfamiliar future, the physicians prescribe him a regimen of deep fried fat, chocolate, and smoking to rebalance him. Although it seemed madness, could the future doctors have had a method based in reason? Eating is a pleasure and pleasure makes your endocannabinoid system activate. When the cells are happy they do good things.

I believe that most of the conventional wisdom and pseudoscience surrounding nutrition is distracting at worst and damaging in many cases. It turns out that we don't need all those carbs from the bottom of the food pyramid pushed upon us by agribusiness. The best available advice currently is to eat a Mediterranean diet but who knows if that will change? Until we know differently, this is what I suggest.

TMT Eating Guidelines

- Get to know the Mediterranean diet components. Avoid excess sugar or carbs, which are glycemic and therefore fattening and try to keep away from processed or factory-farmed animal products. Eat what agrees with your body and energizes you.

- Manage your appetite—keep healthy snacks available to eat like fruit and drink lots of water to suppress ghrelin. But always enjoy your food!

- Favor a plant-based diet—like a "salad as big as your head" or a green smoothie a day.

- Intermittent fasting is good! Although we didn't cover this topic, cell death and autophagy (intracellular waste clearance) are triggered by daily fasting, so if you occasionally skip breakfast and don't eat past 6 P.M., you can get a good 18 hours of cell turnover every day.

CONCLUSION

Why did I write a chapter suggesting that all eating is healthy? Because it is essentially true. Honestly, if we really needed to micromanage our micronutrients in order to be healthy, then we would all be dead within days from forgetting to ingest this or that. There is a lot of margin for error, efficiency, and creativity in your system of digestion and metabolism. From Eskimos to vegans, there is no monopoly on viable eating choices as you don't miss out on certain nutrients.

There is good news when it comes to preventing an old body and sluggish metabolism. Even with "good" or "bad" foods and behaviors, if we maintain high levels of telomerase activity through breathing, mind-set, sleep, and exercise, we are actually able to stave off the changes that cause metabolic slowing.

In the next chapter will touch upon some of those molecules that we do need to supplement. But keep in mind that you will have a very hard time getting sick from lack of those nutrients because they are present in foods and your body will extract them; also bear in mind that you will not benefit and may be damaged from having an excess of them.

Chapter 9

Your Supplements

*Step right up, son. I hold in my
hand the ancient elixir of eternal life!*

Things to ponder:

Why does a lack of vitamins cause disease but a surfeit also cause disease?

What kinds of nutrients are absent from our diets?

Why do all longevity gurus get old and die?

If you had a way to maximize your stem cell telomeres, would you take it?

In this chapter, we will challenge some basic assumptions about supplements and explain which ones are of proven value and why.

It is estimated that Americans spend tens of billions of dollars each year on supplements. Here is a list of the top selling supplements (in descending order): fish oil, followed by multivitamins, CoQ10, vitamin D, B vitamins, magnesium, calcium, probiotics, and vitamin C.

Which of these do most people need because of inadequate dietary consumption?

None of them!

Science shows us that a deficiency of any of them will cause problems, but which ones will enhance healthy functioning beyond a placebo effect when taken in excess?

Surprisingly, the answer is again: none of them.[1]

Of course, you can "supplement" anything, and that is indeed what we should do in many areas, as we've already discussed. Back in Chapter 4, you learned about supplemental and conscious breathing, how it enhances presence, regulates blood pH, and activates your endocannabinoid system by engaging the parasympathetic response. In Chapter 5, you learned how supplemental mindfulness tames your demons and enhances your enjoyment of the moments that comprise your life. Chapter 6 focused on supplemental sleep in the form of higher quality and quantity and how this enhancement of rest engages a myriad of repair and restoration mechanisms in your mind and body. Chapter 7, on exercise, taught how supplemental exercise destroys and rebuilds your body while increasing endorphins, anabolic hormones, cardiopulmonary efficiency, strength, flexibility, and calm. Finally, as you learned in the last chapter, supplementing your diet with more Mediterranean types of foods is thought to enhance telomere maintenance.

So what can a chapter on dietary supplements accomplish?

1. First, we will learn which vitamins, minerals, essential fatty acids, and essential amino acids you actually need.

2. Next, we will critically examine some biochemical pathways that are a little less well trodden. These include trendy new supplements intended to prevent oxidative damage, enhance mitochondrial functioning, and enhance other biochemical pathways.

3. Finally, we will talk about hormonal supplementation, herbs, and telomerase activators.

I don't possess all the answers, but together, we will ask some good questions and acquire the knowledge base to resist blind faith in supplement peddlers.

A common theme in this book that I've returned to again and again is the concept that you already have everything you need within your being and body to optimize your health and to slow aging. As long as you strive for *lokahi* (Hawaiian for balanced flow, discussed on page 107) in all areas of your life, you will thrive.

WHAT'S THE PURPOSE OF SUPPLEMENTS?

From a cynical perspective, a supplement can be defined as something an expert sells you for profit or the enhancement of their pet theory. When I discuss telomerase activators, I confess I am no exception to the rule. We will discuss vitamins, minerals, dietary supplements, fad molecules, hormones, and herbal extracts. I don't mean to suggest that these things are of no benefit, but rather that you as the buyer should always beware, because in the long run, all supplements are subject to debunking for two main reasons that most people don't readily perceive:

1. It is untrue that excess consumption of something that you only need a little of is beneficial. Even sunlight, water, breathing, eating, and exercise can kill you if you overdo them.

2. Telomere/stem cell damage produces aberrations that can't be easily fixed; they are making chromosome-level breaks, causing gene mutation and cellular dysfunction, so the aberrant levels of molecules that we are measuring are the *result* and not the potential *cure* of these problems. Instead of trying to supplement low levels of those molecules, we would do better to replace the damaged cells producing the odd levels of calcium, magnesium, testosterone, CoQ10, and NADH+ that we are measuring.

Let's first step back and get a foundational overview of supplements and all their forms: vitamins, minerals, hormones, and herbs.

Vitamins Are Important Only if You Have a Bizarre or Extreme Diet

There are 13 recognized substances we call vitamins and they were identified because their absences will result in very specific diseases.[2] Vitamins are molecules that your body needs for certain chemical reactions; if you don't have enough of them, unique disease manifestations occur. Your body can only make two of them, vitamin D and vitamin K, and the other 11 must be ingested.

For example, British sailors were once called "limeys," because in the 1850s, the Royal Navy added limes to diluted rum (grog) to supplement vitamin C deficiency and to prevent scurvy, a disease causing the faulty synthesis of collagen.[3] Of the 12 other vitamins whose absence causes known diseases in humans, some of the better-known ones include B1 or thiamine, causing beriberi (discovered in the captive eaters of the 19th-century Japanese navy, who subsisted on polished rice[4]); B9 or folic acid, which causes anemia and is associated with neural tube birth defects; vitamin D, whose deficiency causes bone-deforming rickets; and vitamin K, whose deficiency causes blood clotting disorders.

The truth is that humans have a wide range of vitamin levels in which we operate safely, and they are most often and most easily extracted from a balanced diet. Use your intuition to understand that vitamins are actually like steering wheels for cars. If you don't have a steering wheel, you have a problem steering, but if you have a bunch of steering wheels—that wouldn't improve steering, right? You should also be warned that the fat-soluble vitamins (A-D-E-K) are especially dangerous because they are stored in fat at proportional levels and can build up to toxic levels. In contrast, most other vitamins are water soluble and more easily excreted.

The problem with excess vitamin supplementation is that it is of unproven benefit. Most epidemiological evidence and basic common sense confirm this. In one longitudinal study published in the *Archives of Internal Medicine,* of 38,772 women in Iowa in 1986, 1997, and 2004, researchers found that multivitamin use was associated with an increased risk of dying, compared to those who didn't supplement.[5]

Simply stated: many people were sold (and decided to buy) the idea that just because too little vitamins cause disease, then a surfeit will promote wellness. Wrong! Actually, the opposite of a vitamin deficiency disease, it turns out, is a dangerous vitamin excess disease in every case.

Non-Vitamin Dietary Needs: Essential Minerals, Fatty Acids, and Amino Acids

Essential minerals: To paraphrase Carl Sagan, we may be made of "star stuff," but we aren't literally stars, so it follows that we can't synthesize elements directly and instead have to ingest nearly everything from our diet. Luckily, a balanced diet contains many compounds with the calcium, sodium, chloride, phosphorous, potassium, magnesium, selenium, copper, iron, and zinc that our bodies need. Only people with chronic blood loss from gastrointestinal bleeding or excessive menstruation should need to supplement iron.

An exception that proves this general rule of elemental abundance in most diets is the element of iodine, needed by the thyroid gland. Prior to the iodization of table salt in the 1920s, iodine intake was naturally low in many areas without marine food sources, such as the Great Lakes, Appalachia, and most of Canada. This led to thyroid deficiency and enlarged thyroid glands in the neck (a condition known as goiters).

Essential fatty acids such as omega-3 and omega-6 cannot be made by mammals and must be ingested in the diet. Luckily these fatty acids are present in a wide range of foods such as fish, seeds, nuts, and eggs. The body takes these fatty acids from the diet and assembles larger fatty acids from them that are critical for making all of cells' membranes and also myelin, the fatty insulation covering our nerve cells' axons (the wiring that conducts electrical impulses across distances). Essential fatty acids also are needed to create small molecules that regulate inflammation as well as those happy-go-lucky endocannabinoid molecules.

Essential amino acids are the 9 building blocks of proteins that our bodies can't synthesize. (The other 11 of our amino acids we can synthesize.) Luckily, almost everything you can eat has protein, because all plants and animals use the same biochemistry and the same amino acids to function. It is an unfortunate misnomer to refer to meats as "proteins" because it implies plants don't have protein. False! Of course, if you subsist on a diet of highly processed foods, then the potential exists for extractions of food to no longer possess the natural range of proteins that would be present in living plants and animals.

FAD SUPPLEMENTS AND HOW THEY FAIL

Antioxidants, CoQ10, NADH, Resveratrol, and Probiotics

Some supplements seem to steal the spotlight, including antioxidants, sirtuin activators, mitochondrial function enhancers like coenzyme Q10 and nicotinamide precursors, and the good-for-you bugs found in probiotics. As you've heard again and again—the hype about these supplements is just that—your body is already set up to produce and extract all it needs from a healthy diet.

Antioxidants: What are they? One of the biggest canards in science has been the idea of taking antioxidants to boost health. My opinion is not commonly shared, although the scientific evidence shows taking antioxidants is not beneficial and actually may be harmful, especially in regard to the progression of cancer. Still, knowledge plus dogma has trumped intuition for nearly every person on the planet who accepts the groupthink that antioxidants have been proven to be clinically beneficial.

Oxygen is an oxidant and we need it to live. (That should be your first clue that oxidation is not the root of our problems.) Why would you take an *anti*-oxidant? Technically, *oxidation* just means donating electrons and is always accompanied by *reduction* (or accepting electrons)—it all balances out. In fact, our cellular metabolism and survival depends on these REDOX (reduction plus oxidation) chemical reactions taking place constantly in both the processing of food metabolites in the citric acid (or Krebs) cycle and in the manufacturing of ATP in the 1,000 to 2,000 "bacterial" battery packs known as mitochondria that live in each cell.

To say that oxidation or reduction is good or bad is a fundamental error. That would be like saying that spending money and earning money are bad for an economy. There can be no oxidation without reduction and they both are at the heart of cellular metabolism.

In taking tests in medical school, there was a particularly annoying form of trick question that pertained to two distinct statements that were the downfall of many a student. The answer took the form of: "Statement A is TRUE, Statement B is TRUE, but Statements A and B are UNRELATED." Of course, "unrelated" is not broadly true for anything; it just meant there was no direct causal link and if you made such a link, you'd missed the trick question. Well, let me explain why the story of antioxidants and aging is a myth of the "TRUE, TRUE, but UNRELATED" kind.

It seems that every television news-bit on healthy diets talks about the miracles of antioxidants in berries, broccoli, and kale. I believe that the original claims about antioxidants came from a misinterpretation of why old and damaged cells are spewing out reactive oxygen species (ROS), or electron-grabbing molecules from their mitochondria. People blamed the fire on the smoke. The simpler explanation is that telomere erosion is what causes this phenomenon of excessive ROS. As discussed in Chapter 2, when telomeres shorten, chromosomes combine and the cell detects the improper number of chromosomes, triggering cell suicide or apoptosis through a master watchman enzyme called **p53**. p53 signals enzymes to poke holes in the mitochondria, which are like batteries filled with acid, and the cell thereby destroys itself like the Wicked Witch of the West melting into goo. If you were to show up at the scene of this dying old villain, you might think the smoke arising from the Wicked Witch's body caused her to die, and you might warn young witches to carry around smoke evacuators. You would be giving bad advice. This is the premise of antioxidants preventing aging in a nutshell.

In fact, redox reactions are omnipresent and precisely regulated engines of metabolism. There are ample intracellular antioxidants such as catalase, glutathione, and peroxidase that are efficiently cleaning up after the normal amount of ROS leakage from the mitochondria. The bloodstream is not where most of the greatest potential damage and need for antioxidation takes place; it is mostly intracellular.

As mentioned in the witch analogy, when extremely high levels are pouring out of senescent cells, it is because the cell is trying to melt itself. This is the reason why cancer specialists caution not to take antioxidants when the destructive radiation and chemo are trying to accelerate mutation and p53-driven cell suicide via the thousands of piñata explosions we know as mitochondrial lysis.

To revisit: Do old cells have excessive ROS? TRUE. Do mitochondria malfunction when a cell is old and dysfunctional? TRUE. Are oxidation and primary mitochondrial dysfunction driving aging? UNRELATED.

The bottom line: If you don't believe me, check out the study by the University of Texas researchers who engineered mice to lack two major antioxidants. The rate of mutation and cancer increased but the longevity was unchanged. They concluded that "thus, these data do not support a significant role for increased oxidative stress as a result of compromised mitochondrial antioxidant defenses in modulating life span in mice and do not support the oxidative stress theory of aging."[6]

Are there dangers to cell structures, especially lipid membranes, from oxidative damage? TRUE. Do these dangers increase in aging cells? TRUE. But the ample pathways for antioxidation in a healthy functioning cell mean they are not driving damage but are occurring as collateral damage from the voluntary, late-stage self-immolation of damaged cell popping the piñatas. Smoke from the fire doesn't cause arson, so they are chronologically UNRELATED.

CoQ10[7] and NADH Metabolic Mirages

Coenzyme Q10 (CoQ10) is synthesized in every cell of your body for use in the thousands of mitochondria as an acceptor and donor of electrons for something called the **electron transport chain,** which is an assortment of proteins embedded in the inner membrane that creates a literal battery encased in the walled off mitochondria. A proton excess (or H+) is created with the help of coenzyme Q10 and the subsequent flowing of the protons from outside to inside the inner membrane powers an enzyme called **ATP synthase** that, like its name suggests, synthesizes ATP by oxidative phosphorylation (making energetically charged ATP from depleted ADP and a phosphate) by using the flow of protons.[8]

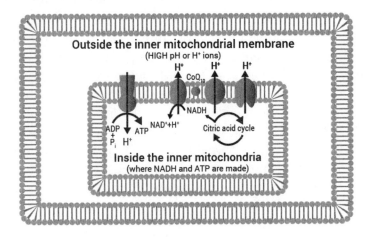

NADH stands for nicotinamide adenine dinucleotide hydride, and it is also an electron-transporting molecule. This is a molecule needed for operation of the citric acid cycle (which makes ATP from glucose and other nutritional sources) and also helps to power the proton pumps that create the battery charge across the membrane that was described above.

Why Taking Them Doesn't Work

While it is TRUE that senescent cells have declining levels of CoQ10 and NADH and it is TRUE that CoQ10 and NADH are essential for metabolic functioning, the decline in CoQ10 and NADH causing aging appears to be UNRELATED. They are simply cogs in the metabolic machine that are readily produced by healthy cells. It is the failure of the cells from a variety of gene mutations that probably leads to declining levels. There are nine genes required to make CoQ10 and they exist in your nuclear DNA, not the mitochondrial genome. Similarly, the gene for making NADH exists on human chromosome 1.

Mitochondria themselves are disposable, simple, and robust. The proteins needed for some, but not all, of their functions come from human protein synthesis, making them true symbiotic organisms. It isn't mitochondria mutation that causes their decline in function, it is the controlling human genes that make up the mitochondrial proteins. The small circular genome of mitochondria does not age like linear host chromosomes, and it contains only 37 genes that encode for only 13 proteins. It follows that human DNA mutation, as occurs with telomere attrition and our theory of aging, is sufficient to explain the one disease with many faces, even a face of mitochondrial dysfunction. Continuing with the "where there's smoke, there's a chance to believe a bogus theory" theme, the dysfunctional mitochondria are like the "smoking gun" of aging and a popular place where discourse goes to die when it comes to theories of aging. But the problem is the victim was murdered by telomere erosion, not gunsmoke inhalation.[9, 10]

If abnormally high levels of ROS and abnormally low levels of CoQ10 and NADH are like wrinkles, gray hair, and bulging stomachs of cells, then ask yourself: Would Botox, hair dye, and liposuction reverse your actual aging? What would? Replacing genetically mutated stem cells with less damaged ones, as your body is constantly doing.

The bottom line: A mitochondrial theory of aging is based on circumstantial evidence and falls apart when viewed with logic and intuition. Avoid antioxidants, CoQ10, and NADH supplements, as they are tantamount to treating arson with smoke evacuators.

Resveratrol

What is it? Resveratrol and the sirtuin story was an unfortunate distraction and a lucrative business model that has hopefully run its course.

It was conjured in the minds of wine aficionados that there was something called "The French Paradox." Somebody came up with the notion that a class of signaling molecules, called sirtuins, that are activated when cells come under stress as with starvation could confer longevity outside of a type of primitive fish. They took a massive leap of faith to say that the one very rare molecule of resveratrol in red wine was what was accounting for the increased longevity of the French via the sirtuin pathway. This would be like saying the reason your team won the Superbowl was because you turned your cap 30 degrees to the right in the fourth quarter and never washed it. If enough people believed it, we would have a lot of dirty turned caps. Well, that is like the story of how sirtuin activators like resveratrol became a credible anti-aging supplement.[11]

Billions of research dollars later, it turns out that the premise of French people having lower rates of heart disease from the minuscule amounts of resveratrol in red wine was bogus on every level: theoretical, experimental, epidemiological, and clinical. GlaxoSmithKline, the unfortunate buyers of a sirtuin research company called Sirtis, abandoned their $720 million venture due to toxicity and a wide range of failed experiments.

The "if this, then that" reasoning that is the sirtuin/caloric restriction story was a Sisyphean boulder pushed up a hill by greed, groupthink, and conjecture. Do sirtuins play a role in enhancing cell survival under the stress of caloric restriction? TRUE. Does resveratrol in very high doses activate sirtuins? TRUE.

Is activating sirtuin pathways a natural mechanism to combating aging? UNRELATED.

Taking resveratrol to stop aging makes as much sense as taking a sponge bath to get better at swimming. Even though caloric restriction toughens cells by putting them into distress mode, is it worth torturing your cells to try to reap a benefit? This is the antithesis of the endocannabinoid system. There is no positive evidence to support this will impact longevity but plenty of evidence to suggest taking resveratrol or other sirtuin activators is harmful. A major drug company had $720 million worth of reasons to want this to be untrue but you might still believe it because you heard people you respect repeat it enough times on television.

Probiotics

What are they? These are friendly bacteria that you ingest or insert that restore or rebalance the good flora over the bad. While it is true that we constantly harbor bacteria in our lower gastro-intestinal tracts, skin, and lower female reproductive tracts, the potential benefits of probiotics are lowest in the form they are commonly used: eating. Like the vitamin story, aberrations in the natural balance of friendly bacteria are rare. Shifts away from friendly flora are often produced by antibiotics or cleansers that induce extinction events; this allows for opportunistic newcomers to take hold, causing skin infections like MRSA (often pronounced "mersa") or methicillin resistant Staph aureus, infectious diarrhea known as pseudomembranous colitis, and vaginal infections known as bacterial vaginosis.[12]

The fact is that the friendly bacteria that you purchase at the health food store can't even survive the stomach acid and digestive enzymes without some protective encapsulation. Another problem is the rapid and efficient transit through the sterile small intestines means there is nowhere to host them. Research has consistently failed to demonstrate that they live in our relatively sterile small intestines. As bacterial occupants of the colon, the lactobacilli that you buy at the health food store and ingest are unstable and insignificant in numbers.

Is there a benefit to lactobacillus ingestion in some clinical cases? Yes! Is this because the lactobacilli survive and sustain themselves in our gastrointestinal tracts? No. Chalk it up to the placebo effect, which is very real, or to some unclear bacterial homeopathy. Having some ingested lactobacilli survive to your colon is doubtful, but even if it occurred, it would be like a drop of perfume in a septic tank.[13]

Decades of research in humans suggest that although there are lactobacilli above the stomach (in your esophagus and mouth) and in the distal portion (last third) of the small intestine, they do not set up a stable permanent residence like the lactobacilli of the vagina. Furthermore, the contribution of intestinal lactobacilli to disease and wellness is poorly established. I know I may sound crazy because so many people believe it probiotics, but don't kill the messenger. We have knowledge and intuition to guide us.

Fecal transplantation: A related practice of "fecal transplantation" has taken the notion of probiotics to an absurd level. The idea that your colonic bacteria (not lactobacilli) can be optimized by putting someone else's poop up there strikes me as pseudoscientific except in cases of rare colon colonization with something known as *Clostridium difficile*, which is usually produced by antibiotic use. Do you want to feel really disgusted? It turns out that 60 percent of your feces by weight is composed of bacteria! Considering that, in otherwise healthy people, fecal transplantation seems like trying to improve the smell of my three-day-old garbage by swapping it with a bit of your three-day-old garbage. As with supplementation with vitamins, minerals, antioxidants, and everything else, the body's natural system of hosting bacteria is robust, efficient, and almost never needs meddling from us.

There is an exception that proves the rule of foolishness when it comes to probiotics. In the case of the more common vaginal flora shifts resulting in an amine or "fishy" odor, common problems that shift the acid-producing flora to unfriendly species are use of soaps, douching, and the presence of alkaline fluids such as semen, saliva, and blood. In those cases, a vaginal antibiotic cream can be inserted, or you can use a dilute vinegar solution to restore the acid milieu and competitive advantage of the lactobacilli that have temporarily been overwhelmed by the alkaline-loving competition.

Hormone Supplementation

The sex hormones of **estrogen** and **testosterone** wane as we age. It's the process of aging, probably via damage to stem cells from telomere shortening, that causes people to produce less sex hormones as they get older. Of course, a precipitous drop in hormones comes with female menopause and the cessation of ovulation in the late 40s, whereas the gradual decline in men has been referred to as "andropause."

Athletes of all ages use anabolic steroids to increase muscle mass, but they come with many risks, such as acne, baldness, aggression, masculinization, testicular atrophy, and menstrual irregularity.[14] Human growth hormone (HGH) is popular as an expensive and off-label injected supplement for would be anti-aging aficionados and body builders. There is some possibility that HGH can enhance cancer formation, so care should be taken. Other risks include fluid retention, joint and muscle pain, carpal tunnel syndrome, and high blood sugar.[15]

Voluminous research indicates that supplementation with estrogen for women and testosterone for men, at physiologic levels, benefits older people, as we will discuss in the next section. This is not to say you are fixing the root problem of stem cell aging, but sex hormones do play an important ongoing role in cell signaling and health maintenance and therefore replacement benefits probably do outweigh the risks.

There was a case-control study from Korea showing that users of estrogen replacement had longer telomeres.[16]

There was also a study from the NIH showing that treating people with telomere-shortening diseases showing that the synthetic hormone, Danazol (a synthetic steroid), improved telomere length in 92 percent of participants. The study was halted due to ethical concerns. It was working too well to withhold from half the subjects, and the researchers were surprised at the level of effect.[17]

There are strong logical and epidemiological arguments for hormone replacement, especially bioidentical human sex hormones like estrogen and testosterone. We qualify this with "human" because much of the research was based on horse estrogens in urine (from pregnant mares, to be specific, hence Pre-mar-in, or one of the most researched and prescribed versions of estrogen supplementation). The benefits of hormone supplementation are many but must be mitigated by the exaggerated fears of cancer promulgated by medical and public health officials. The decision of how and whether to replace sex hormones is best individualized with the help of a trained physician.

Many of the benefits of hormone therapy—better sleep, enhanced sexual and exercise performance, higher rates of energy, improved mood, and increased health markers—are similar to the effects of telomerase activators, suggesting that they also act by similar mechanisms. Restoring hormonal balance is something that impacts every cell of the body and the case can be made that the risks of cancer have been overstated and that the benefits far outweigh them, especially when it comes to restoring the myriad of pathways that we need to function at our optimal telomere repair efficiency.

Does supplementation of sex hormones contradict what I'm saying about not needing supplementation? Yes and no. Of course it would be preferable to prevent stem cell deterioration and drop in hormonal production, but since these hormones are global and powerful mediators of cell signaling and overall function, supplementing them is not akin to adding some incidental extra metabolic gears to a broken machine as with CoQ10 or NADH.

Herbs Are Bioactive Cocktails

Then there are rich herbal medicine traditions such as Chinese Traditional and Indian Ayurveda that use different systems of conceptualizing health based on pathways, energies, and relationships that don't yet fit into the reductionist system of the Western scientific method. Are there potent, scientifically reproducible pathways that are modulated by the component molecules in them? Most definitely. Many of the most potent pharmaceuticals Western medicine uses originated from the plant pharmacopeia. Do we understand them? Not by a long shot.

When supplementing with herbs, it is important to consider several factors. Safety and purity are critical and when possible, you should seek out certificates of authenticity that show organic farming and lack of pesticides and harmful contaminants like lead, mercury, and infectious agents. Secondly, you should learn all you can about the experimental and theoretical benefits of the supplements you are taking, leaning toward those that are GRAS ("generally recognized as safe"). Finally, you should experiment with how you feel, one at a time. There are countless reasons why a placebo or biochemical effect might vary from person to person, which are completely opaque—so trust your intuition and listen to your body.

Herbal Telomerase Activators

My intuition about telomeres being a fundamental mechanism of aging has been confirmed from my taking a telomerase activator as my sole supplement since 2007. In 2008, in response to the requests of my patients, I became the first physician outside the TA Sciences company to "prescribe" them, and since then, I have learned from my most successful patients that incorporating diet, exercise, sleep, and mind-set provides even more synergy and faster improvements in health than merely taking the supplement alone.

My personal and clinical experience involves herbally extracted telomerase activators. There is an interesting extract from a Chinese herb that I began to take in 2007 called TA-65, which was discovered by a Menlo Park biotech company called Geron; the telomerase activation was validated by U.S. Patent No.

7,846,904 in 2011. Since 2007, the molecule in TA-65 is the only supplement that I have taken, and I have helped thousands of others enjoy the benefits, placebo or otherwise.

Unlike the cocktails of thousands of molecules in traditional herbal medicine, this molecule is the purified, single molecule from a Chinese herb known as *huang qi* (aka astragalus) that was thought to enhance life force (qi is pronounced "chi"), increase longevity, and improve immunity. Like the THC from marijuana, this TA-65 molecule may be one of the molecules in the huang qi that was doing the "heavy lifting" of telomerase activation that is at the heart of my telomere/Telomere and Stem Cell Theory of Aging.

Is huang qi in traditional Chinese medicine believed to enhance qi, longevity, and immunity? TRUE. Does this huang qi extract of TA-65 enhance telomerase activity? TRUE. Does TA-65 from huang qi improve energy, stem cell survival, and reverse immune senescence via telomerase activation? TRUE, TRUE, and LIKELY RELATED.

The U.S. Patent application affirms that this single molecule extract indirectly enhances telomerase activity. My personal experience with this as well as my clinical practice since was my introduction to holistic health and the gateway to my development of my Telomere and Stem Cell Theory of Aging.

Evidence shows that TA-65 doesn't directly increase gene transcription of the telomerase enzyme. It appears to work through increasing endocannabinoid signaling although it doesn't create a feeling of being "high." In doing so, it creates an adaptogenic effect, meaning it takes you into a state of better flow, balance, and healing—just like breathing, meditation, sleep, and exercise.[18]

My own experience with taking a telomerase activator supplement has convinced me that there are real benefits; within three months, I lost 15 pounds without any dieting or exercise; sleep improved, as did my prediabetic condition, hypertension, and fatty liver. Could this have been a pure placebo affect? Certainly. But I have many instances of unsolicited signs and symptoms of getting younger that there could be much more at work.

In general, energy, sleep, mood, and skin improve along with a reduced need for reading glasses and darker hair pigment.

Concerns over an increased risk of cancer do not appear experimentally or clinically validated in my interpretation of the literature and in my experience. In fact, cancer may be a disease primarily of stem cells so it follows that keeping those healthy with telomerase activation will lower the rate of cancer formation, its severity, and maintain the ability of those cancerous cells to kill themselves or be eradicated by the immune system. The best proof of a telomere and cancer connection was published in the *Journal of the American Medical Association* in 2010. It prospectively followed 787 participants, of whom 92 (11.7 percent) eventually showed clinical cancer. The shortest telomere lengths were associated with higher risks of getting cancer and more severe types and these risks decreased with increased telomere length.[19]

I'm currently one of the few evangelists in both the areas of "telomerase activation medicine" and "adaptogenic medicine and physiology." Adaptogens, by definition, make some folks eat or sleep more and others eat or sleep less; the effect depends on how far from normal you are currently deviated. I have had countless insights while producing my video seminars, lectures, and blogs based on my patients and my research. To learn more about my clinical experience with adaptogens and telomerase activators, check out my YouTube channel, "drpark65."

WHAT ARE COMMON NUTRITIONAL SUPPLEMENT DEFICIENCIES?

To put it succinctly, there are no common vitamin or supplemental nutrient deficiencies in the developed world as long as you iodize your salt and have access to fruits, nuts, vegetables, and fish. If you were a dark-skinned person living above the Arctic Circle, then you might get rickets from vitamin D deficiency owing to poor light absorption. If you were a sailor in the 17th century without limes in your grog, then you might develop scurvy. If you were a WWII British prisoner of war in a Japanese Imperial camp in Burma eating only polished rice, then you might have developed beriberi. But we have to assume that these conditions are not easy to reproduce in a person with access to a variety of foods—that's most of us.

That said, vegetarians should supplement with vitamin B12 because their dietary intake is often too low, causing a type of anemia or low blood count. Another subgroup that can be at risk for nutritional supplement deficiencies are people with obsessive eating habits who voluntarily consume the same processed foods daily (for example, instant ramen). Food authenticity and variety is important; a recent study found that nearly 60 percent of the average calorie intake comes from ultra-processed foods like sodas, cereals, frozen meals, instant soup, and so on.

Simply stated: dietary extraction of essential minerals, fatty acids, and amino acids should not be a problem for most people. Having said that, just to be safe, we have taken to protecting unborn fetuses with folic acid (to prevent neural tube defects), calcium (to build bone), and sometimes DHA (an omega-3 fatty acid needed for brain development).

Supplementation of calcium has become standard procedure and there is some evidence to suggest that it may be associated with decreased mortality. Having said that, excessive intake is dangerous, and in fact, calcium and phosphorous serum levels are tightly regulated by the parathyroid gland.[20] If the bone cells are not storing calcium because of telomere-induced damage to those stem cells, no amount of calcium supplementation will change that.

There are a variety of conditions that cause thyroid deficiency, and they can even include stress related to adrenal gland exhaustion. If you feel tired or abnormally cold, have a slow heart rate, have dry skin, and are constipated, there is a possibility you might have a low thyroid hormone level, which can be diagnosed and treated fairly easily or possibly improved by iodine supplementation. If your thyroid cells are senescent and damaged and your pituitary/hypothalamic regulation is faulty, perhaps some regimens such as intermittent fasting and curcumin will help clear the damaged cells so that balance can be restored.

Finally, magnesium supplementation has also become trendy because people believe they have a deficiency. Although studies show that magnesium has been associated with a higher mortality, an interesting study showed that you couldn't even raise your magnesium levels with oral supplementation. In a placebo-controlled trial of young men, the only change between taking magnesium and a placebo was the amount of magnesium in the urine, not the blood. This again suggests that the cells are functioning properly, like when the "bad cholesterol rises" from underutilization of cholesterol. The problem lies in damaged stem cells and their abnormal behavior because that is ultimately what determines the blood levels of magnesium.[21]

WHAT DOES TELOMERE SCIENCE SAY ABOUT SUPPLEMENTS?

What Supplements Are Best to Take?

If you have been paying attention, the list is very short. If you have limited meat consumption, vitamin B12 is a good idea. Calcium supplementation appears to be helpful in small doses. If you don't add iodized salt commonly, then iodine is also needed, but it is plentiful in seafood, yogurt, and turkey breast. In older folks, the benefit of sex hormone replacement is strongly supported by the evidence. Finally, there are cutting-edge supplements like telomerase activators that might slow the very process of cellular aging, which may be generating the oxidative toxins and aberrant levels of CoQ10 and NADH seen in the mitochondria of aging cells.

We need to learn as much as we can and experiment cautiously with the powerful and potentially dangerous substances in herbal traditions. Many of them have been adapted into Western medicines, like foxglove decocted into digitalis, a potent cardiac rhythm drug. That said, many herbs are generally recognized as safe and some of them have entourage effects (meaning the complex effects of the whole substance not entirely understood by the sum of the parts). A classic example is the emergent use of marijuana versus pure THC. Some allege that you can't just extract THC (tetrahydrocannabinol) and expect the same benefits as assimilating the many other substances in marijuana, like CBD (cannabidiol), which have had proven benefits in treating cancer, for instance.

Telomerase Activators

There are studies looking at telomerase activation and inhibition from various supplements. Because of the methodological challenges and lack of general consensus, I will refrain from quoting them in the interests of time and limiting confusion. To date, the astragalus derivative I mentioned above has the most clinical experience and peer-reviewed research. Suffice it to say that it might be worth your effort and expense to see if the enhancement of all the TMTs while taking a telomerase activator can be reproduced in your life to create an "upward spiral." Although other experts openly tout telomerase activation by the lifestyle interventions mentioned in this book, they balk at recommending telomerase activating supplements. So it is up to you to decide whether supplementation with telomerase activating properties are something you want to try.

Adaptogens Work with Your Body, Unlike Pharmaceuticals

Adaptogenic physiology is based on the idea that existing systems of your entire body are always promoting balance and flow. An adaptogen is something that produces different effects in different people depending on their physiology; they might make one person sleepy and other alert. Their effects depend on what is out of balance for you.

Western medicine is largely developed from billion-dollar blockbuster molecules often reverse engineered from plants that are intended to block pathways that normally function. If we take the major classes of high blood pressure medications as an example, they are blockers of the sympathetic nervous system, blockers of water absorption, blockers of calcium channels that allow arterial constriction, and blockers of the kidney and adrenal functioning via the hormones that allow vascular constriction and sodium retention. The unfortunate consequences of drugs is that they can cause untoward side effects and even harm because they isolate and inhibit systems that are working to achieve natural balance.

What if I told you that high blood pressure is just caused by aging of the arteries and is actually an adaptation to get the blood pressure to where it needs to go, like kinking a garden hose to control the water flow? That doesn't mean it can't be dangerous or shouldn't be treated; it just means that pharmaceuticals are treating the harder problem of remediation in isolation, instead of prevention through higher telomerase activity and maintaining stem cell youth.

All of this is not to suggest that you can't benefit from drugs when needed. If you have T cells infected with HIV, bacterial pneumonia in your lungs, intestinal parasites in your colon, or fungal organisms in your brain, your native immune system may not be scalable, robust, or trained enough to fight them before they overwhelm you causing permanent disability or death.

If you are going to supplement with anything, do some research into forms of traditional Ayurvedic or Chinese medicine and find a safe version of whatever tonic you feel you need. Then experiment, one herbal adaptogenic supplement at a time, and trust your intuition. Be careful to do your research before taking them, however, as they can have powerful effects and even interact with medications you take.

CONCLUSION

If we consider optimal health to be the presence of balance and flow in the absence of disease, then rather than focusing on supplementation, we should probably just eat a variety of naturally derived foods, preferably borrowing heavily from the Mediterranean diet, as discussed in Chapter 8. "Let food be thy medicine," as Greek physician Hippocrates said. The take-home point of this chapter would probably be: save your money and lay off most supplements by just eating a healthy, diverse diet. If you want to experiment with one supplement, I would recommend astragalus derivatives, which have proven telomerase activating and adaptogenic properties. By keeping the stem cells happily dividing, dying off when damaged, and slower to mutate, you are likely to benefit from all of the other TMTs if you do. That's what I practice and that's what I preach and so far, so good as I enjoy a healthy life at 50 years of age, free of disease and the need for medicines.

But enough about me. In the next chapters, we will explore a topic of much greater interest and perhaps the reason you have taken this journey of learning to this point: let's talk about *you* and how you can truthfully assess how you're doing with regard to the TMTs and maximizing your telomere and stem cell integrity for a better life.

PART III

THE TELOMIRROR PLAN IN ACTION

Now that we have mastered all six TeloMirror Tools of breathing, mind-set, sleep, exercise, diet, and supplements, let's put them to use in your individualized plan. This will require some self-examination. Instead of a one-size-fits-all prescription, let's find out what best suits you. But before we do our self-assessment, let's recap what we have learned thus far.

1. There are thousands of studies linking better telomere integrity and by inference, higher telomerase activity, with higher functioning of all the TMTs. They are simply mirroring how efficiently your natural healing is taking place.

2. Being "unstuck" or in a state of *lokahi* (balanced flow) appears to be the foundation of adaptogenic wellness and it probably relates to endocannabinoids,

mind-body awareness, and eliminating habits that rob us of mindfulness, gratitude, and presence.

3. All the TMTs work together synergistically, like cylinders in an engine. If you treat your sleep apnea and do a gratitude list before bedtime, you will have better breathing, more positive beliefs and more efficient healing. If you exercise, you release anabolic hormones, endorphins, and endocannabinoids to feel better and sleep better, avoiding obesity and daytime fatigue. We can't always be "firing on all cylinders," as they say, but let's at least get them turning the camshaft in the same direction.

4. You, your organs, your cells, and their telomeres already possess the ability to maintain health and wellness! As Dorothy from *The Wizard of Oz* learned, there never was any magic in the man hiding behind the curtain. You and I have always had the heart, the brain, the courage, and the means to return home.

I think the best possible news in all of this is that you have the means to reverse aging without the need for a prescription, a thought leader, or a scientific paper to validate you. You can take positive steps now because telomere research just mirrors back what you have likely known all along: wellness is within. You now have the information to be your own expert on staying young. Now you understand how your cells are naturally endowed to help you succeed in maintaining your optimal health and happiness.

So, let's take the next two chapters to look within and design a personalized framework that will yield the greatest joy, flow, and presence so that you can remain as healthy as possible while we await science to master stem cell replacement technology.

Chapter 10

What Do You See in Your TeloMirrors?

The only thing that makes sense is change.

This chapter addresses the "why" and "what" of making changes. We will discuss both why we should bother changing and why inertia (resistance to change) exists. Then we take inventory of what you are actually doing in all the six main areas. The "who" and "where" of are fairly self-evident; *who* is you . . . and *where* is in your thoughts, beliefs, and actions. Finally, the "how" is for Chapter 11, where we will use the data from our inventory to craft some changes for your daily routines.

Before we start, let me take the pressure off you and me both by stating what I truly believe in the form of this manifesto:

> We shouldn't expect to feel amazing or even be optimized all the time. There is no perfect way to do anything so thankfully, your mind and body are forgiving and adaptable allies. Making mistakes is how we learn and we can only aspire to make new ones rather than repeat old ones. We believe that science and subjective experience can be forged into practical wisdom for better living.

This book was intended to be a "quick start" guide for some critical aspects of your life. My goal is to help you achieve comprehensive yet practical mastery of cell biology and genetics, breathing, consciousness, sleep, exercise, diet, and supplements—all of which will help you to live a long, healthy, and happy life. It may not always have been easy to comprehend, but if you've tried, you've received a plethora of information to inoculate you against being mesmerized and misled by experts and groups that sell you on ideas of uncertain staying power and veracity. With the notable exception of my emotional meta-tagging theory of consciousness, everything I have presented herein is rather fundamental orthodoxy. I hope you will consider rereading chapters as needed,whenever you are faced with a new paradigm. Some hot new recommendations might not jibe with the real physiology, and now you are able to question them.

So, what was the big idea of this book? That there is one simple, intuitive, and science-based unifying theory of aging and disease based upon telomere erosion in stem cells. The rate of erosion determines the rates of mutation, cell dysfunction, and depletion of healthy reserves, but thankfully, science suggests that erosion can be mitigated by healthy habits under your control.

Even though there are thousands of studies showing that telomere dysfunction is related to poor health, shorter lives, and nearly all forms of disease and aging, experts resist my simple interpretation as stated. Those experts make a living off perpetual quests and wars, and if we had a simple and treatable cause, it would be an unmitigated disaster. Scientists who study aging hope for a simple theory in the same way oil companies are passionate about providing free solar energy to everyone.

I say that the association between telomeres and diseases associated with aging is causal, but there will be billions of dollars, tens of thousands more studies, and perhaps decades of time wasted before this simple idea becomes orthodoxy, if it ever does at all. Isaac Newton treated the apple and the moon the same when trying to derive equations to describe gravity. But Newton didn't have mortgages and private schools to pay for.

YOU ARE THE EXPERT

Let's revel in all the wisdom you have acquired thus far. You now know that genetics are not destiny. If you are alive, chances are most of your genes are fine, but that doesn't mean you aren't susceptible to new mutations in stem cells caused mainly by telomere erosion. Being alive means that you have agency to protect your stem cells, activate telomerase, and preserve your telomeres. Following all the TMTs will help you to live happier, healthier, and longer.

Here is a brief recap of the tools you have at your disposal:

- The first TMT is **breathing**, which takes in oxygen for cell respiration, balances pH, and clears carbon dioxide. Breathing also engages the relaxation response, and therefore protects your telomeres. Make sure to practice mindful breathing and adopt practices in your posture and sleep that will help you best leverage this tool.

- Memory and beliefs are built using emotions, and so reframing your **mind-set** to be centered on gratitude and befriending the demons in your mind are keys to maintaining balanced flow. Practicing a positive mind-set lowers stress and improves happiness and health—all of which enhance how your cells, telomeres, and telomerase work.

- You discovered that **sleep** is organized into 90-minute cycles, and each cycle provides different types of dream states, brain activity, and body restoration processes that operate in a structured and purposeful way. Getting a nightly eight and a half hours or more of sleep enables the healing required to repair your spirit, mind, body, and telomeres. Good sleep hygiene and practicing gratitude before bed are strategies that help you get the most from sleep.

- **Exercise** should be safe, challenging, and fun. You know to focus on "playing out" instead of working out. You also have a deeper understanding of how exercise is a process of overstressing muscle fibers, connective tissue, and the cardiovascular system, which coaxes your body to adapt by growing stronger and more flexible. Moderate regular exercise enhances cellular regeneration and will extend your quality and quantity of life.

- Food is a pleasure to be enjoyed in a guilt-free, yet mindful, way. **Eating** strategies are best individualized. Focus on managing appetite and favoring a plant-based Mediterranean diet, whenever possible. You learned to avoid highly processed foods and about the consequences of highly glycemic foods.

- **Supplements** are not needed, except physiological doses of sex hormones, iodine, or vitamin B12 for vegetarians. Telomerase activating supplements and other adaptogenic herbs may help you to stay healthy, happy, and live longer. See page 250 for a review on the supplements I recommend.

When I was a practicing ob-gyn, I was astonished by the frequency with which I heard the phrase "I know my own body" from women who were sometimes misinterpreting certain mechanics of their physiology. These knowledge deficits ranged from reasons for midcycle spotting and irregular bleeding to declining fertility with age, the causes of vaginal infections, and many other misconceptions. Despite my anatomical disadvantage, I had a more accurate understanding of their bodies from education and clinical experience. My point is that intuition without knowledge leads to mistakes, while blindly following expert opinion is a poor substitute for field-tested knowledge. It takes both—intuition coupled with fundamental knowledge—to lead you toward personalized wisdom. We are all humans who breathe, think, sleep, exercise, eat, and take supplements. But you are now in a subset of humans who "know their own bodies" in these six areas. Each chapter was structured in the same way: purpose, physiology, pitfalls, telomere science, and optimization of each of these areas. Learning to run a diagnostic program on these cylinders of your engine will be the focus of *this* chapter. In the next chapter, you'll work on a personalized plan that can endlessly adjust the engine's efficiency.

If you understood the previous chapters, you are ready to unlock the wellness within you. It was probably uncomfortable to rethink antioxidants, "bad" food, sleeping just six hours, and the authenticity of identity, but discomfort is the price of growth. Just ask the immortal lobster! Discomfort, for the lobster, is a signal to molt and grow a bigger shell. If your subconscious goal was to reinforce what you already believe, then you have only cheated yourself, like the man who asked the question in my lecture and then left before my reply (see page xi). Without embracing the new paradigms offered in this book, you will not experience the full benefits you could.

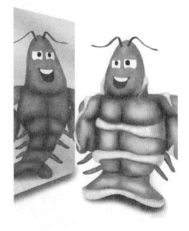

The ever-expanding scientific literature (of which I've only shared a small fraction) suggests that these six cylinders (or TMTs) of your life are strongly associated with healthy telomeres and lower incidence of disease and dysfunction. My unified theory suggests that telomere maintenance will keep you younger and healthier, but studies are not necessarily translatable to your real life, and so that will be the goal of this and the next chapter. To that end, I want you to engage in an honest and careful inventory of yourself. However, before I have you take a self-inventory, it's helpful to understand why change is desirable and why it is so difficult to implement.

SELF-TRANSCENDENCE = MORE HAPPINESS

Abe Maslow, an American psychologist, is well known for his theory of human motivation, "Maslow's Hierarchy of Needs," which was published in 1943 and is still taught in sociology and management programs fairly universally. Maslow studied high-achieving American college students and prominent individuals like Albert Einstein and Eleanor Roosevelt in the early 20th century, and he used his findings to construct a pyramid that attempted to identify the fundamental human needs, from most basic to most sophisticated. His conclusion was that people who are preoccupied with the most fundamental needs such as food, thirst, sex, and safety can't focus on higher-order needs such as belonging and love.[1] Near the top of Maslow's pyramid is self-esteem, and at the very top is his concept of self-actualization (defined as the ability of a person to realize his or her maximum potential).

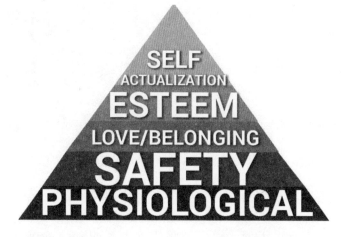

Despite the triangular imagery, the hierarchy of needs isn't a reverse champagne tower that fills from each level on up. All needs can be filled or go empty from time to time, and at different rates. Later in life, Maslow added a capstone to his pyramid, including another phase or level—that of self-transcendence (having a higher goal, purpose, or meaning in life that generally serves others).[2, 3]

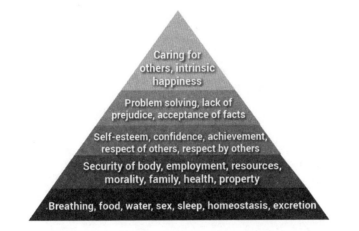

Self-transcendence is important because it recognizes that service to self is unsatisfactory when compared to living in service and harmony with a larger world. Let's say that you've already achieved many of your needs and are accomplished in terms of the "checkboxes of life," such as a home in a safe neighborhood, career, financial security, a supportive family, friends, and good health. You may feel pretty self-actualized. Still, even the most accomplished people can feel empty if they are not giving back, serving others, and/or contributing to the betterment of the world. Self-transcendence feels good because it reaffirms the truth of living: that we are all interconnected and are most powerful when we are aligned with a joyful purpose.

What Does Self-Transcendence Have to Do with Keeping Your Telomeres Healthy?

The resistance to creating a bigger shell to inhabit or creating a more efficient engine for living comes down to a lack of a sincere desire for self-transcendence. As scary and inhospitable a neighborhood as one's own mind can be, we sabotage change because we believe the subconscious demons whispering to us that the misery we know is more manageable than the unfamiliar bliss we could be creating. If we transcend ourselves too quickly, the demons of ego, ambition, and scarcity might feel threatened.

When we focus on possessions, identity, and experiences, we often don't see that those are mere avatars for the abundance, connection, and sensations that are inexorably available to us in every moment. Dorothy of Kansas was always home and her companions always possessed the heart, courage, and smarts that they were seeking. People who believe that the programmed voices they've empowered to run their lives are providing a truthful representation of reality will have little impetus to find a new and higher level of fulfillment from self-transcendence, however incremental or monumental the change.

If you find yourself committed to a pattern of thinking that goes something like—

> *I consistently exercise five times a week, take my vitamins and fish oil capsules. I always sleep six hours a night and if I sleep more I feel groggy and unproductive. I never eat sweets and I have a glass of red wine to increase resveratrol, so I don't really think I can do much more to improve my health and longevity.*

—then you really haven't embraced this book. You are comfortable in your current lobster shell and will age normally, but we all know what normal aging looks and feels like, and how it ends.

To change your course, it's vital that you believe in things that most health experts don't make money from, such as laughter, play, dance, creativity, community engagement, service to others—all those things are going to make you a happier, more grateful, and more telomerase-active person.

How would this pattern of thinking look? Someone ready to molt out of the old lobster shell of beliefs and behaviors and grow a new one might be thinking—

> *I'll give it a try. It all seems plausible. I'm going to eat better foods and take adaptogens before sleep with a snack. I will read instead of watching TV or my device and plan my bedtime to allow a minimum of eight and a half hours of sleep. I'm going to do my top 10 gratitude list each day, set the thermostat to 76 degrees, sleep in the secondary bedroom naked after hugging*

my partner and telling them something I love about them. I will keep a mouthwash spray by the bed, and after I naturally wake up, I will lie there with eyes closed and positively visualize my day. I will stretch and meditate for 15 minutes, shower, and enjoy a nice blended green smoothie. On the way to work and all day, I will try to be grateful, observant, and focus on deep, mindful breathing. I will smile at most everyone I see. I will eat small portions of delicious foods and drink plenty of water. I will get to my exercise, yoga, or dance class and fully commit to it. I will enjoy a sit-down dinner with my loved ones and be genuinely interested and encouraging about their days. I will not watch the cable news or watch whatever happens to be on. I'm going to text or call a sibling, child, or parent to tell them I love them.

Someone who isn't quite sure about change might think—

I didn't want to snack before sleep because experts say that it makes you fat, and I was afraid the adaptogens would keep me up all night. Instead, I watched the news and got anxious about terrorism and radicalized politics. I was so worried that I did an Internet search, and found more news that suggested things were worse than I imagined, which kept me up way past my bedtime. I forgot to do the silly gratitude thing, and that may be why I had a nightmare about having to fight some crazy fish monster. When the alarm rang five and a half hours later, I hit the snooze, but I really didn't want to go back to fighting the fish monster, so I dragged myself into the shower, sighing deeply as I noted the bags under my eyes. I turned the TV on again while I stuffed some food into my mouth as the cable news continued the awful story from yesterday and everyone in the house scrambled to get out the door. On my way to work, I was so angered by the idiots driving around me that I didn't notice the kid on the bike that I almost hit. At work, I wanted to take a nap, but instead I answered e-mails, gossiped, and drank coffee. I ate something I usually don't eat, by myself, which made me feel guilty, so I left work early to go to exercise *class. I found myself distracted during class and pulled a muscle. When I got home, I had a glass of wine to relax and fell asleep next to my partner, who was griping about something awful on the cable news. The fish monster was gone, but it was replaced by a three-headed serpent. I woke at 3 A.M. in a cold sweat with my partner snoring and the TV still blaring. I surfed the Internet for an hour and looked up places to retire on less than $1,000 a month.*

The first person is giving the program an honest try and building confidence through an "upward spiral." The second person never really wanted to incorporate change, because he or she is too sleep-deprived, anxious, and scarcity-minded to transcend suffering.

Why Would the Lightbulb Really *Want* to Change?

Here is an old joke pertaining to change: "How many psychiatrists does it take to change a lightbulb?" The punchline: "Only one, but the lightbulb has to really want to change." As any psychotherapist will tell you, most people make a game of pretending to not know what their problems truly are. People create stories and conjure scapegoats because it is just easier. If you tell yourself, "I only have time to sleep six hours," or "I have to eat whatever my spouse does," then you might be resistant to change. If you found a recommendation in this book annoying, that might point to an area that especially needs fixing. It all boils down to sleeping more, being grateful, consciously breathing, exercising regularly, eating Mediterranean more frequently, finding time to laugh, sing, and dance, and considering adaptogens.

> *Young souls learn to accept responsibility*
> *for their actions.*
> *Mature souls learn to accept responsibility*
> *for their thoughts.*
> *And old souls . . . learn to accept responsibility*
> *for their happiness.*
> — **Mike Dooley's** Notes from the Universe

If you tell yourself, "I'm doing everything experts tell me to do," you may be a young soul. If you embrace the idea of gratitude and mindfulness, you may be a mature soul. But if you want to find maximal bliss through mastery and wisdom, you may be an old soul.

The inability to exorcise the personal "demons" that consensually run our lives is why some schools of psychiatry have experimented with hallucinogenic drugs in the most severe forms of mental illness, such as addiction, depression, or post-traumatic stress disorder (PTSD). The thinking here is that psychedelically induced depersonalization can momentarily allow you to see yourself as you truly are because you are able to experience your consciousness from outside of the experience of identity and ego investment. In a drug-induced, highly depersonalized state, you can use mirror neurons in a heightened way to truly observe yourself. Inability to self-transcend is no accident. We are complicit in enabling our dysfunctional behaviors and limiting beliefs because deep down, the demons have convinced us that they are there to help us survive.

For example, a person berates her partner because her ego feels threatened by emotional engagement and she might be acting out behavior internalized as a child. Conflict feels like intimacy, but it degrades the quality of the relationship. As another example, a person is always getting sick and letting everyone know. Instead of taking steps to be healthier, the demons or subconscious malware in these examples use conflict or a sick-person role to receive attention without risking vulnerability.

So your challenge, no matter how self-aware you believe you are and no matter how much "shadow work" you've done to examine the darker reaches of your psyche, is to do something bold and creative. We can all vividly envision the awful, and many of us spend far too much of our lives doing precisely that. What is much harder to imagine is the amazing and wonderful future that we could have. The answer to "Why is change hard?" is that we tend to be lazy and fearful. The answer to "Why change?" is that we can always do better and we know it.

As we plan better habits and lives, remember that "believing is seeing," not the other way around. You have to believe there is a bigger lobster shell in your future. So, the question I pose is, "Are you ready to be surprised by how amazing, healthy, and happy your life can become?" If your answer is yes, read on.

DAILY SELF-INVENTORY

Quantum theorists and statisticians know that the mere fact of observing something ALWAYS changes the outcome. If you are doing a precise daily inventory of how you breathe, think, sleep, exercise, and eat, you must accept that the results are going to be biased because you are judging yourself as you record. That's okay. Judging while you observe is ultimately how you are going to find your wellness within. Like balancing on one foot, *lokahi*—or being balanced while flowing with change—is the optimal state of being for healthy, happy humans.

Nevertheless, before you begin to introduce change, I encourage you to take a telomere wellness holiday for now. Document, without judgment, how you typically live your life as if you had never read the previous chapters of the book. As much as possible, this means that I want you to conduct your life for a week just exactly as you usually would with regard to breathing, mindset, sleep, exercise, eating, and supplements. Once you've done this, you'll have established a baseline from which to evaluate and improve going forward. You'll use this data and your current lifestyle patterns in the next chapter to craft some changes that will get you functioning at a higher and more blissful level.

How It Works

Most of our lives are organized around weeks. Sunday-to-Sunday is how we tend to count them because of work, school, and calendars. Once you have accumulated eight straight days of TMT self-inventory, you will compile your data and look for patterns in the next chapter.

You'll find a "TeloMirror Self-Inventory" checklist on the next page. On the page after that, I've partially filled in a checklist with some sample responses; your responses will vary.

Print out eight copies of the checklist on the next page, and fill it out each day, either as you go through your day, or at a quiet time every night before bed. Start on a Sunday and end the following Sunday.

TeloMirror Self-Inventory

(Day _____)

Sleep (best recorded when you first wake up):

- Last thoughts before my last night's sleep: _____

  _____

- Time I went to sleep: _____
- Time I awoke: _____
- Total hours slept and # of 90-minute cycles:_____
    - ~4½ hours or less equals 3 cycles or less
    - ~6 hours equals 4 cycles
    - ~7½ hours equals 5 cycles
    - ~8½ hours equals 6 cycles
    - ~9½+ hours equals 7+ cycles
- Sleep Notes (e.g., trouble getting to sleep, awakenings and what woke you, and any vivid dreams): _____

  _____

Conscious breathing or meditation done today: _____

_____

Exercise done (times and type):_____

Eating (with whom and what I ate):
- Breakfast:_____
- Snack:_____
- Lunch: _____
- Snack:_____
- Dinner: _____
- Snack:_____

Supplements taken: _____

Notes on any memorable conflicts, self-loathing, anger, or anxiousness:

_____

Notes on any memorable bonding, blessings, achievements, gratitude, optimism: _____

Quality of life assessment:

Give yourself a grade of A to F for this day with respect to
- EnJOYment _____
- Authenticity_____
- Presence_____
- Productivity _____
- Gratitude_____
- Self-compassion _____

Ed's Sample TeloMirror Self-Inventory

(Sunday, May 4)

Sleep (best recorded when you first wake up):

- Last thoughts before my last night's sleep: *"I need more money,"* *"My health is deteriorating"*

- Time I went to sleep: *11:30 P.M.* *(although I was reading for 30 minutes from 11 P.M.)*

- Time I awoke: *8 A.M.*

- Total hours slept and # of 90-minute cycles: *8½ hrs = 6 cycles*

- Sleep Notes (e.g., trouble getting to sleep, awakenings and what woke you, and any vivid dreams): *I read some scary article about economic collapse. I woke to pee once at 6 A.M. Dreamt about being chased by a tiger who ate my leg.*

Conscious breathing or meditation done today: *I didn't think about breathing*

Exercise done (times and type): *gym for 1 hr (20 minutes elliptical and 25 minutes weight training)*

Eating (with whom and what I ate):

- Breakfast:_____
- Snack:_____
- Lunch: _____
- Snack:_____
- Dinner: _____
- Snack:_____

Supplements taken: _____

Notes on any memorable conflicts, self-loathing, anger, or anxiousness:
_____

Notes on any memorable bonding, blessings, achievements, gratitude, optimism: _____

Quality of life assessment:

Give yourself a grade of A to F for this day with respect to

- EnJOYment _____
- Authenticity_____
- Presence_____
- Productivity _____
- Gratitude_____
- Self-compassion _____

SELF-COMPASSION AND BALANCE

As a final note to this chapter, let's talk about the last item on that scorecard. Self-compassion is hard for many people. As I briefly mentioned in Chapter 5, this stems from a narcissistic delusion. Let me describe where I first realized this truth. I was once at a seminar where the facilitator asked people to look into handheld mirrors and say something nice to themselves. People found it consistently difficult to do, and that's when it occurred to me that the reason stems from a sort of narcissism.

The way we would talk to others is more kind than the way we talk to ourselves. If you have ever been in a relationship with an exquisite narcissist, they will tell you, "I thought you knew all the great things I feel for you, so I only gave you the negative feedback!" What if I told you that the inability to be kind to yourself represents the same kind of false lack of separation from yourself that a narcissist with poor boundaries feels toward family members? It is because you fail to perceive the separate and individual dignity of yourself that you talk to yourself so shabbily! It is the same mirror neurons that we need to feel empathy and introspection (creating an abstract version of us).

In contradistinction, a person who is taking hallucinogens or who has stopped fully identifying with her ego and its attendant demons will not have the same trouble thinking good things about herself (or others, for that matter). So, self-compassion is like putting on your oxygen mask at 30,000 feet. If you don't put yours on first, you'll be unable to help others with their masks. Once you feel compassion for yourself, you can feel it for others and even for the demons running most of your thinking.

When we have self-compassion, we will tend toward balance. As we shift to a new equilibrium, it may often seem like three steps forward and two steps (or more) back. This isn't rocket science or brain surgery; it is horseshoes and hand grenades. Growing accustomed to a new and better homeostasis, whether it involves diet or exercise or practicing self-compassion and C.A.R.E. techniques (see page 115), will take some practice. Don't worry about occasionally swinging to extremes or backsliding; simply try for a middle pathway. Our point on the horizon is a sustainable integration of a more pleasant and mindful way of living. Self-compassion is appreciating when you are doing the best that you can by taking responsibility for your actions, thoughts, and happiness. It does not mean playing a static story where you are always the victim and everything is someone else's fault. If you cast yourself as the victim, you lose agency and power. You can't always change what happens but if you don't try to change how you react to it, you have no hope of transcending your perceived problems. You are the guru. Your method is simply the intention of better living. Life is your teacher.

CONCLUSION

We want to change because we want to optimize and we resist it because we are lazy and fearful. If you accept the manifesto that we aren't trying to be perfect, just better, then it's time to put knowledge and data into service. How can we start to make some tweaks and experiment with better optimizing the cylinders of our natural healing? That is the subject of the next chapter—tuning up and learning to constantly monitor and adjust the engine.

Chapter 11

Your TeloMirror Tune-Up

I'm so happy now I can barely stand myself.

And . . . we have now, finally, officially mixed the dueling metaphors of mirrors and engines. At this point, you should have eight self-inventory pages from the last chapter (if you don't, see the inventory on page 236). Let's take a look at what you've learned about your lifestyle from your week-long inventory before you consider any changes you might want to make.

The first week allows you to take a somewhat honest look at how you run your life. As you begin to incorporate changes, you can use the same methods to perform continuous and weekly evaluations and adjustments.

COMPILING THE DATA

As we "mine the data," try not to obsess over some statistical methodology, although you are free to make spreadsheets and do that if you feel it will be helpful. It's horseshoes and hand grenades, remember? Just lay all eight pages out, Sunday to Sunday, and take it all in. It should be pretty fresh in your mind and you might be amused, surprised, and occasionally delighted by what you find.

SLEEP REVIEW

Is Sleep Deprivation Driving Your Mood and Productivity?

The first thing I want you to do is see if there was any correlation between lack of sleep the night before and the quality of life axes of EnJOYment, Authenticity, Presence, Productivity, Gratitude, and Self-Compassion the following day. If you had less than six hours of sleep, you might find some bad grades; if you had nine or more of sleep, you might have had a good one.

Last Thoughts before Sleep

I hope that you will try the "Top 10 Things I'm Grateful For" practice because it may be one of the most powerful tools in this entire book. Your thoughts and beliefs are so personal and seem so real, but they are all just stories that you tell yourself, and stories can be told with many different voices, spins, and morals, can't they? Some people will find it difficult to even hear their own thoughts; it's like asking fish to describe the feeling of water. But if someone next to you could actually hear the way you think and tell stories, you probably would sound a lot like Gollum, the mumbling sociopathic degenerate hobbit from *The Lord of the Rings*. You can fake it during the day, but the world of dreams is harder to control, and whether it will be demons or angels that shape your memories, beliefs, and narratives is somewhat under your control.

If you recalled and recorded your dreams in the morning, then try to correlate them with your last thoughts before going to sleep. It seems rather obvious, doesn't it? The thing you worry about or feel blessed about appears in your dreams in some form or other. What kinds of themes emerged from your last thoughts? If you are like most people, the last thoughts you hosted might have been worries from watching the news, worries about money, worries about loved ones, or worries about getting enough sleep. You really need to refrain from all that worrying because it only sows seeds of anxiety for bad dreams, which form bad beliefs, and then you cultivate a garden of grief that awaits you during REM sleep and procedural memory formation. You can see now that this is a particularly dangerous habit. As previously mentioned, there is a very good reason they say "never go to bed angry with your partner," and now you understand it. If you were practicing active gratitude and presence throughout your day, the strength and emotional meta-tagging of the day might be somewhat gentler; if you blame everything on a convenient target like your spouse, your procedural memory will create more stories around that narrative.

I realized the importance of this sleep incubation from telomerase-activator-using patients. They just make you more intensely you, which can be a good thing or not so good, depending. Some patients reported wonderful dreams and others reported nightmares, although if they let their subconscious make a miniseries out of the turmoil, even the ones with stressful dreams often rose to whatever challenges they had conjured. The consistent difference was in the thoughts and paradigms people focused on just before sleep. When you focus on gratitude before sleep, you get to choose what genre of movie your dream mind will be cueing up that night. Do you want to watch the horror movie or the musical comedy? Think of yourself as a suggestible child about to drift off to sleep. Who would you rather have tucking you in? Maria von Trapp (the lovely ex-nun played by Julie Andrews in the movie *The Sound of Music*) or Annie Wilkes (the kidnapper/"number one fan" played by Kathy Bates in Stephen King's *Misery*)?

Take a moment to cross out any negative pre-sleep thoughts on your pages. I want you to strike a line right through them. Now, for each negative thought, write out an antitoxin belief from abundance and gratitude. Change thoughts such as "This neighborhood is dangerous" to "I am grateful that I have not experienced crime." "I don't make enough money" becomes "I am grateful that I can pay my bills." Worry about loved ones becomes "I am grateful that my family is able to pursue their goals and learning resilience." A worry such as "What if I don't get eight and a half hours of sleep?" can be transformed into "I have gone to sleep plenty early enough and if I need to, I can always take a nap tomorrow."

Daily Homework—Choose Wisely the Seeds You'll Sow

You can draw a mind map, write a list, type a spreadsheet, or make up a jingle about your favorite thoughts before sleep. I don't know what you are worried about but you certainly do. Construct some antidote paradigms and positive affirmations to supplant those worries. I know that there is always room to invite some outright blessings into your consciousness before sleep as well. Practice the "Top 10 List of Things I'm Grateful For" before sleeping so that it becomes a nightly ritual. You get to start with the annoying stuff, reframed with gratitude, then you get to keep it real with material blessings, then acknowledge the people you cherish, finally ending with something unique about yourself, the most deserving and desperately in need of your compassion of all.

Early to Bed?

Did you understand the assignment of recording bedtime? If you went to bed at 10:30 P.M. but were on social media for an hour, your bedtime was the time you actually fell asleep: 11:30 P.M. You should never watch TV news before sleep because it gets a direct subconscious pathway into your psyche, and most of it is pretty terrifying and of questionable veracity. Instead, listen to or play some music, read a book, make love, or take a soothing bath before you turn in. Time spent in bed, not sleeping, decidedly does NOT count as sleep time.

Did You Really Need That Worm?

What time did you wake up? Many people with work and school commitments tend to wake up at the same time every day. That's a good thing for your circadian rhythm. But if your schedule showed irregularity, like 4½, then 6, then 8½, then 6 hours, you need to take a look at how you conduct yourself. Always plan your bedtime around an ideal amount of sleep time. Start your work earlier on the front end and see if you can't adjust the morning so you can sleep in. I know that we all have commitments and situations pop up, especially when you have children and rigid job schedules. Nevertheless, you can usually make adjustments to try to keep your sleep blocks sacrosanct.

Staying up all night produces work of inconsistent quality and adversely impacts your productivity and circadian rhythm afterward. Here's a really obvious suggestion that many people ignore: if you have to wake up early, then go to bed earlier or at least take a nap the following day.

Total Hours/Cycles?

If you were paying attention, you will notice the total sleep will generally organize into 90-minute cycles, although the sixth cycle and onward may tend to be shorter, like just an hour's duration. That is how it generally works although there can be lot of variance. If you have the luxury of waking up naturally in the morning, you can keep track of what your sleep cycles tend to be after the usual 90-minute blocks of the first five cycles. And remember, just because you are awake after seven and a half hours, that doesn't mean you can't have a more blissful day by indulging in one or two more sleep cycles. We may be slaves to wages, commutes, and other duties, but if you really think about the hours in a day we spend doing mindless frittering, there is usually stuff you can curtail in favor of precious sleep.

Many people in modern life have adapted to a mere six hours (four 90-minute cycles) of sleeping. That is the bare minimum. If you are operating on four and half hours (three cycles), you may feel pretty awesome about yourself, have an awesome body, and have awesome friends and an awesome lifestyle, but you may also be suffering from a sleep-induced Dunning-Kruger effect. You are so diminished from sleep deprivation that you don't even know you are impaired. As they saying goes, if three people tell you to sit down at a party, you are probably drunk. I have yet to meet the person operating on four and a half hours of sleep who can just smile in the face of outrageous fortune the way that I can on 10-plus hours of sleep.

If you are operating on five cycles (seven and a half hours), you are probably caught on some hamster wheel of adult living. You are going to school, taking kids to school, working a 9-to-5 job, and generally have your nose to the grindstone. My advice to you? Go to sleep an hour earlier—please. Your telomeres will thank you and you may be preventing Alzheimer's, obesity, and all the other diseases by doing so.

If you are getting six cycles (eight and a half hours, as the sixth cycle can tend to be shorter), congratulations! You are now doing the very least that your mind and body needs to repair those telomeres.

If you are getting seven or more cycles (nine and a half plus hours) then you are going to enjoy better telomeres, a longer and more blissful life, and make those around you so much happier by just being around them. Sure, you may be sacrificing quantity of wakeful hours, but you might enhance the quality of them with respect to joy and productivity.

Homework: Make the Time for Sleep

Go through your records and try to account for why you got to sleep too late or woke up too early. If you had a late night partying, did you make sure you could sleep in? The circadian rhythm is a form of homeostasis and will tend to remain constant. Now that TV shows are streaming on demand, did you really need to stay up late? As you balance your nightly rituals, your morning commutes, and whatever extenuating circumstances you have, try to always make room for a nine-hour block of time.

Notes: Troubles with Sleep

If you had trouble getting to sleep, was there caffeine within six hours of bedtime? Was your room a comfortable temperature and free from sensory distractions? Were you anxious about something? Did you wear comfortable jammies or sleep naked? What was your sleep position? Go back to Chapter 6 if you need to review how to optimize your environment and how to use your pillows or neck rolls.

If you woke up once per night to empty your bladder, that is good and normal as long as you didn't have trouble getting back to sleep. Sleeping with a full bladder is bad and causes an increase in your blood pressure. Drinking water before bed is fine unless you have an enlarged prostate or inefficient bladder emptying due to antihistamine sleep medications. It is a good practice to keep a glass of water and some mouth spray or breath strips on your nightstand to maintain hydration and kissability. The most important thing to consider when you wake up is that you mustn't engage your conscious mind by checking e-mails or thinking about tomorrow—stay in the primitive parts of your mind, like stumbling out of your tent and then back into it after drinking beers. Just because you are marginally awake, that doesn't mean you should wake up and start your day before getting optimal sleep. Kill that idea now before it kills you!

If you had vivid dreams, take note of their content. There will be answers to unresolved issues there and your dreams often have a high correlation with the last thoughts you had before sleep, whether positive or negative.

BREATHING AND MEDITATION REVIEW

If you are like most people, you didn't likely do any conscious breathing or meditation last week. That's fine. It's only your first week. If, upon awakening, you lay in bed with your eyes closed visualizing your day for 45 seconds while consciously breathing, that counts as a mini-meditation. If you were able to sit quietly and breath consciously while meditating, that counts too. If you went to yoga, did cardio, or did 4-7-8 or box breathing in traffic (see page 82), that also counts. In fact, if you spent any time at all thinking about your breathing, count it and keep it up. Mindful breathing is an instant magical transporter to the present moment. In the present moment, there isn't any room for regret or worry. In the present, you are just alive and consciously breathing connects you to how abundant and calm things can always feel, even amid the chaos of living.

Meditation is a pleasure that most people cannot imagine, but for many it becomes a positive addiction. Find a technique of sitting comfortably, fingertips touching, eyes mostly closed, and thoughts freely flowing as you consciously breathe. There are many focused and purposeful meditation techniques, mantras, and visualizations for you to discover or invent. Don't try for anything in particular but instead be a good listener, like a good friend. Have fun and remember this is a dedicated time to C.A.R.E. Clear the clutter of ego identification, audit those automatic thoughts, reframe with gratitude, and enjoy the present moment.

Review the breathing techniques for calm, focus, and increased energy we discussed in Chapter 4. Remember that whenever you feel anything untoward, you can immediately and positively restore balance and presence by breathing deeply and mindfully. It's like having those ruby slippers that Dorothy always wore. They can't come off unless you're dead, just like breathing can't stop unless you're dead. So just click your heels and breathe and in no time, you'll be right back at home (in your heart). The flying monkeys and wicked witches can wait a few moments while you prepare to do battle.

EXERCISE REVIEW

This should be fairly easy to report, as most people go somewhere, like a gym or a class, to get their exercise. But if you decided to walk six blocks or take the stairs, count it! If you were on vacation and went skiing, surfing, or biking, count that! If you decided to go dancing, you can count the heck out of that! If you did some calisthenics or mindful stretching, you can count that too.

What did you notice about exercise? Are you ever skipping it from laziness or other commitments? Don't forget that a few minutes of push-ups, leg squats, and sit-ups are always available to you. You have to use it or you lose it and your body needs that creative destruction.

Reflect upon what physical activity made you most joyful and that will guide you to increasing the time and space for those activities. We want to "play out," not "work out," remember? Did you take the stairs before lunch? Did you walk a friend's dog? Did you dance in your underwear to that one song that always gets you dancing at weddings? Good for you! Keep it up because there are a million ways to choose to be active and use that amazing body you still possess.

EATING REVIEW

If you noticed, there are six meals on your checklist although you may have only partaken of three. When it comes to managing hunger, insulin, blood sugar, and energy, six is better. For many people, there will be four to six hours between meals. That means you will get hungry, tend to eat more at lunch and dinner, lose focus, and become "hangry." What kind of snacks should you have? As long as it isn't a ton of food, anything is fine. That's right, a little rib eye or cheesecake is fine; enjoy with gusto and lots of water. If you really want to be "good," you can have fruit, nuts, vegetables, a small salad, or a bit of your next meal in advance.

As you examine the meals you had, what patterns emerge? Are you a creature of habit or did you like variety? Was convenience a priority or did you dutifully prepare your own meals? Was there a decision to eat healthy at the expense of enjoyment? How often did you end up eating alone and was it by choice? We are not judging your choices, but by directing some consciousness toward these questions perhaps you can imagine some changes that will increase enjoyment, quality, variety, and meaning?

Did you engage in so-called "emotional eating"? You wouldn't shame yourself for sleeping in if tired or for shivering if cold, so don't start a shame spiral for a bit of ice cream in response to stress. Just be mindful that carbs found in sugary foods, breads, and pastas are going to be quite glycemic, so treat them with respect. As you start to engage in an upward spiral of looking, feeling, and acting more blissfully, your tendency to binge on glycemic foods should decrease.

SUPPLEMENTS REVIEW

Did you take your physiological replacement hormones, such as estrogen, testosterone, or thyroid replacement? If you are one of the many people who take lots of multiple supplements, please consider stopping them all and then adding them back, one at a time, to see what the effects are. First, you must read up about common effects to help interpret subtle changes and how they can affect you. Some are best taken at a specific time of day and some need to be taken with fatty food or on an empty stomach. After you have taken your supplements individually and know how they impact you, you can start to add them back in combination or stop them.

If you believe in them, did you take adaptogens? If you did take an astragalus derivative or another adaptogenic herb, was it at night, during the day, or around the clock? Did you notice enhanced dreaming or brief awakenings as most people report on adaptogens? Did you have a better mood and less need for caffeine? Did you recover from injury and exercise more quickly?

REVIEWING THE SPEED BUMPS OF LIFE

Conflict, Self-Loathing, Projecting Anger, Anxiousness

Let's take a look at stuff that triggered you. Did speed bumps tend to cluster on days when you had poor sleep, a bad attitude, no exercise, ate poorly and infrequently, and were tense? If your neck and shoulders ache, you may not have taken a cleansing breath all day.

What events or thoughts produced conflict, self-loathing, anger, and anxiousness? For each of these, I want you to ask three questions (R.A.J., if you need a mnemonic):

- Was it REAL (or mostly in my head)?

- What was the ANT (automatic negative thought) that I assigned to it, and which of my ego demons typically uses that tool?

- What is the JUDO MOVE (reframing with gratitude) that I can summon the next time this happens?

For example, a customer calls and complains that you didn't do something right. He is mad, and you feel defensive, angry, and then guilty.

- Was it real? "Yes, I dropped the ball."

- What is the ANT? "I am bad at what I do," says the *you're-not-good-enough demon.*

- What is the JUDO MOVE? "I am grateful for feedback because it's an opportunity to grow. I make mistakes like anyone else, but I am less likely to make that mistake again now."

You can use the supreme R.A.J. technique on all forms of conflict (the word does mean "ruler" or "king" in Indian languages, after all). If you do so, you may find that the disappointment, conflict, anger, anxiousness, and most negative emotions trace back to a form of self-loathing. If your ego expects certain things of you and others and feels it isn't being rewarded, it feeds the demon chatter. If you are grateful, despite and even because you make mistakes and face challenges, then negativity can't find resonance with you. To paraphrase Anaïs Nin, we don't see the world as it is, we see it as we are; so fix your perceptions, and you fix your projections. How you choose to emotionally meta-tag everything matters—it determines your story and how you experience life.

Bonding, Blessings, Achievements, Gratitude, Optimism

What wind was beneath your wings? Take note of the improvements in relationships you had, the unexpected delights, the goals achieved, the gratitude you felt, and the moments of unbridled hope. The more you focus on these things over discernment and scarcity, the more light you invite into your life.

Did you find that on good days, everything seemed to go your way, like you were "on a roll"? Perhaps you will note that you slept well, had nice dreams, ate well, exercised, and connected with everyone in a positive way. I'll bet you were breathing well and relaxed. That is what happens when you "fire on all cylinders" and your endocannabinoid system is kicked in.

People taking adaptogens tend to report being in a state of balanced flow, or *lokahi*. Unless they are accustomed to this, it is quite noteworthy. They report that things that used to trigger them don't bother them like they used to. They notice a high frequency of positive coincidences or synchronicities. They have good focus yet are open to what is happening in real time. In a fractal sense, as our cells flow and experience good balance, so do our organs, their functions, and our experience of life.

Truthfully, I don't know if the "law of attraction" is really what accounts for enhanced positive experiences while "high on life." This magical interconnectedness and flow of energy is omnipresent by definition and that way of being is what small children have to unlearn by being taught to label, discern, and judge, ostensibly for their own socialization and protection. I believe that infinite opportunities for connection, joy, and synergy can't find resonance with us when we are generating fear, scarcity, and robotic interactions. A butterfly wouldn't land on a hot barbeque grill when it can rest on a nearby flower, right?

Barring any disguised allegory about the primacy of the Hero's Journey and Chaos Theory, it is possible that the "Hokey Pokey" song was a spurious explanation of "what it's ALL about." For most of us locked into a subjective reality of feelings, perceptions, and judgments, our quality of life is truly what it's all about.

As you look over last week's pages, take note of how you graded your quality of life in these broad areas. I hope you did so honestly. Our hope is that what once passed for a B will soon feel like a D as you learn to optimize your health and bliss and set higher standards for your state of body and mind.

Enjoyment

Did you enjoy yourself on this wonderful day? If you were living IN joy, you probably did ENjoy yourself. You deserve an A grade. If you were miserable, then you should start looking inside yourself for the cause. But "how can we enjoy when everything is so serious and important to survival?!" our demons ask. We answer by wondering just how real any of those imagined tigers were and how close to pouncing on us they actually were.

Nietzsche explained in his parable that people evolve in stages: first, as children, they are like camels, and the greater the load, the stronger a lion they will become when they wander into the desert of adult life. But the lion must work to slay the dragon covered in "thou shalts" so as to transform back into a child, experiencing the world on its own joyful terms. Be childlike now, before it's too late, because there is no defeating a dragon if you believe what's written on its many scales.

Even in the darkest and most powerless moments, take comfort in knowing that you always have the choice of how you react and where and how we will encounter joy. If you don't believe me, read *Man's Search for Meaning* by psychologist Viktor Frankl, who wrote about the ways in which he and his fellow concentration camp prisoners reacted differently to the same horrifying conditions in concentration camps. We always have a choice on how we interpret life so as to become fully self-actualized lions and then self-transcendent children. The secret to restoring telomeres and joy can be found in mastering breath, emotions, regeneration, movement, and eating food and other magic herbs.

Authenticity

Were you true to yourself today? Were you unafraid to just be yourself and let others see and feel who you truly are? If you resisted the temptation to agree with people just to get along, give yourself an A! You should be proud because most people live their entire life wearing a mask of consensual conformity.

That is never to say that you should just be an offensive jerk with no manners. I don't believe in personality disorders or claiming to be "on the (autistic) spectrum" for most people. I think folks feel more or less inclined to use the mirror neurons and thoughtfulness depending on how much they care to do so given the circumstances.

Authenticity might mean you smiled to get some advantage if you're that kind of person. Hopefully, authenticity means you smiled because you were happy to be with that person. But ideally, you smiled because you were happy to be alive and that is the kind of warmth that no one can easily resist.

Presence

Were you focused and aware throughout the day or did your thoughts stray toward regrets of the past or worries about the future? Regrettably, for most of the denizens of the spaceship Earth, most of their consciousness is spent outside of the present in daydreams of longing, regret, and ego-tripping.

Think about how you were breathing during anxious times; it probably wasn't all that good. Remember that your breath is like clicking those ruby red slippers that bring you right back to what is happening now, both in your head and around your body. Practice being present by using mindful breathing as often as you can. Secondly, work on being present with your emotionally burdensome thoughts by using the C.A.R.E. or R.A.J. techniques. Finally, work on being present for other people by feeling what they are conveying, rather than just trying to prepare your redirect or your trump story in response.

They say that we, as socially interconnected beings, only need a few things to feel good: touch, eye contact, validation, and a smile. If you were able to provide those things for people today, give yourself an A! If you were able to be present with nearly everyone you encountered today, you get an A+ and a gold star! You have significantly improved the world on that day and should feel powerful and proud.

Some say time is like an arrow, so it follows that "the present" is as elusive as expecting a still frame to represent a movie. In contrast to that point of view, I think it is possible that your present can be expanded in both directions using the power of consciousness, so as to render time an illusion, if we consider the matter deeply. You see, we always change the past by remodeling its emotional meta-tagging and changing the stories around that. The future will be entirely experienced under the influence of the imagined future. Let us choose wisely which new demons we allow into our ever-expanding presence. How? By allowing ourselves to feel, to reveal, and then to heal whatever negative emotions we created and to feel, reveal, and then seal whatever blissful ones we conjured.

Productivity

You don't need to complete complex projects, but did you make progress that will get you closer to your goals? If so, great! Hard things are hard and that is why we procrastinate when it comes to them. The fact that you did something positive is wonderful and a sign of a true hero or heroine.

If you closed a chapter and actually realized a goal, then celebrate! If you took a leisure day and didn't get a darn "productive" thing done, congratulations! Rest is a part of the process of achievement, so celebrate your complete lack of forward progress on this day and give yourself a counterintuitive A! That may confuse the heck out of those demons and their automatic negative thoughts (ANTs) so much that they may consider taking up residence elsewhere.

If you spent time sharing presence with people in an authentic way, then this was also being productive. Your relationships require nurturing and friends, coworkers, lovers, and family are just as deserving of your attention as your "real work." Don't create a false dichotomy between work and social productivity, because deep down, you know they both require your joyful and authentic presence. Hmm. We're starting to see a pattern in the quality of life axes. Just as with the six TMTs, the quality of life axes seem to be working toward the same goals, like the cylinders of an engine.

Gratitude

This is the big one. Did you feel it? Did you express it to someone? If you did, did it transform your relationship to a higher level? Give yourself an A! An attitude of gratitude means your cherish and feel honored to be connected to this world and its beings; it is the wisdom of knowing that suffering is not by design but rather by choice and that the choice is always from a misguided desire to resist change. The first three items in the "Top 10 Things I Am Grateful For" practice are reserved for things that really made you feel bad. It is perfectly normal to feel bad but it is unhealthy to not take responsibility for your actions, your thoughts, and your happiness that can be found by doing the J in the R.A.J. technique (the judo move of gratitude).

Self-Compassion

How was your negative self-talk today? Did the demons run the show? That's okay. They are serving some purpose and if you want to know why you welcomed them in to help run your show, you need only ask. Meditate or dream on it, and expose those little goblins with the flashlight of pure consciousness and love. If you managed to think some nice things about yourself, then give yourself an A!

If you need to feel self-compassion in the midst of despair, try to get outside yourself à la Ebenezer Scrooge from *A Christmas Carol*. Imagine you died yesterday. Now use your imagination and visit the people in your life. Are they happy that you are gone? You are a miraculous, brave, important, giving, and divine presence for them all. There is not another being more deserving of love than you.

On the daily TMT inventory, we saved the best for last when it comes to self-compassion. As the study from Spain looking at telomeres among Spanish Zen meditators showed, longer telomeres were associated with being younger, being unafraid to try new things, and a high level of self-compassion. Even if you are a horrible person, doing horrible things without remorse, there can still be room for self-compassion as you have lost your connection to the divine and have chosen a darker path in life.

Strive for self-compassion, not self-delusion and self-aggrandizement. Listen to your heart and your internal moral gyroscope will always bring you back into balance. You are doing the best you can with the demons you have invited to help run your life. You just have to coax them into behaving a little more like angels.

YOUR STRENGTHS AND CHALLENGES

If you were able to complete the inventory for last week, you now know a bit more about how your six TMT cylinders are functioning and how your six quality of life axes performed. What if we could optimize and combine the telomere-enhancing behaviors with the six areas of enjoyment, authenticity, presence, productivity, gratitude, and self-compassion? We could be purring along in a 12-cylinder luxury vehicle!

Spend some time with your eight days of data and refer back to some of the earlier chapters and their recommendations. In which areas could you enhance your telomerase by attending to optimization? Look at your comments, the dreams, the grades, and then seek out the associations that your intuition may find. Now that you have knowledge and a means for meaningful self-evaluation, you are truly on your way to becoming your own health guru! To paraphrase Swiss psychologist Carl Jung, he who looks outside to experts, dreams and will be misled; but he who looks inside with self-knowledge and mastery, awakens and escapes the suffering of time.

So after digesting what the state of your TeloMirror Tools are reflecting back at you, it is time to construct a guideline toward the true alchemy: creating wellness from within.

SCHOOL OF LIFE: CONTINUOUS IMPROVEMENT

Instead of weekly, start referring back every night to the day's inventory and then make a conscious effort to gently correct your homework. You can use red pencil and gold stars if you like. If you went running, had healthy snacks of leftover salmon, and meditated for 15 minutes today, give yourself a star or a smiley face on each of those line items. Now take that pencil and cross out the negative things, and suggest more positive versions. Instead of writing, "you only slept six hours, you idiot," write, "try for eight and a half hours." If you skipped your afternoon snack, print, "keep some nuts at work." If your notes indicate that you felt anxious before sleep, write a gentle reminder to "do the top 10 gratitude list" in the last thoughts before sleep section.

In time, your ability to run the self-inventory will become so automatic that you will do it without pen and paper! If you can learn 26 letters of the alphabet as a six-year-old, you can remember these critical 16 inventory items: thoughts before sleep, time to bed, time of waking, hours slept, meditation, exercise, meals, negative things, positive things, supplements, enjoyment, authenticity, presence, productivity, gratitude, and self-compassion. If you focus on these areas, your life and telomeres can only improve and it will be time to trade up to bigger and bigger lobster shells. Hopefully, you have a nice teacher and the positive comments and stars are more common now that you have been correcting your self-inventory homework for a while.

As with anything, the key to creating positive habits is repetition and insight. The truth is, all your usual behaviors, beliefs, and habits were serving mixed purposes that can be understood and then transcended. It isn't a good or bad thing that you want to achieve instead of being complacent. Getting to know how your psyche works requires continuous self-assessment, revisiting the daily TMT inventory, and checking in with your intuition and meta-consciousness. Don't just seek to control action or thought; seek to control your happiness by radical self-compassion and inviting change.

I suggest that you continue to print out the self-inventory and keep them in a binder. You can also paper clip each week together, and add a new, one-page weekly summary self-inventory that sums up each week, and then attach it to the front. For example, **Week 1: Jan 1 to Jan 8.** You can start to compile a lot of data and might even start to compile a monthly summary as well. Feel free to graph your results. Feel free to just stop if you think you've got it handled and to revisit if you need a tune-up.

If you are living a blissful life, check your inventory. If you are struggling, check your inventory. If you don't know if there has been any change or improvement, just go back to week one and see what life was like before you consciously tried to make some changes.

I didn't want you to do a two- or three-week inventory because it seems like a lot of work rather than fun and therefore you probably wouldn't be compliant. Your goal is to consciously observe, modify, and improve according to the principles in this book. Since every night is a natural boundary between the next day's adventures, it seemed logical to construct your self-assessment around a daily inventory.

If you are forgetting exactly why I recommended eating six times daily, or sleeping nine and a half hours, refer back to Chapter 10 to refresh and rededicate yourself to the core beliefs and the rational choices that emerge from them. We can backslide and even fail, but never give up. You are never going to stop breathing, sleeping, thinking, exercising, and eating; but you can always optimize these areas to enhance your wellness from within.

I recommend taking a few minutes to do the wellness self-inventory every night until you have nothing but good habits left and everything is automatic.

CONCLUSION

Congratulations! You have created new telomerase-activating routines that are now running your life! You don't have to take my word or the word of any expert now. You have the knowledge and the personal experience to see what works best in your life.

They say that it takes about 21 days to cultivate new habits, but these new "habits" should never be unconscious routines; rather, they should allow for continuous improvement. Yes, you can use smartphone reminders to remind you to breathe deeply. I'm sure "there's an app for that." You can prepackage lunches and snacks. You can sign up for exercise and dance classes. The possibilities are infinite and there is nothing but upside when you learn to embrace the positive lifestyle habits that not only do a body good, but help you feel good as well. Your happiness is your responsibility and I hope you are better able to find it after reading and practicing what is in this book.

If you care about living a healthy, long, and happy life, I hope you will never go back to unconscious breathing, automatic negative thinking, sleeping as a waste of time, avoiding exercising, mindless eating, and wasting money on supplements. Everything in this book is scientifically and practically valid despite what expert-endorsed recommendations might have lodged in your beliefs.

You have been given the ability to tune up your six-cylinder engine of telomerase activation and the other six-cylinders of life quality. Don't worry why researchers may be misinterpreting the reasons why telomeres are short in people with poor lifestyles. By acquiring knowledge, you have taken a big and practical leap beyond mere reductive science toward inductive wisdom and mastery of your life. You will "know your body" better than I or any other doctor or expert could. Enjoy your adventure of self-discovery, empowerment, and wellness that will be mirrored by your telomeres.

Finally, please try to worry less. Experts will warn you that if your health is good, you don't ever want to retire; you want to work until you don't feel like it anymore and then find another call to service. I believe that if you can remain relatively healthy for a little while longer, there will be significant advancements to mitigate and reverse whatever aging has already taken place. I hope that the next and final chapter will encourage you to persevere. In it, I will explain what really causes aging and how a few simple technologies could make aging voluntary.

Chapter 12

The Future Is Ageless

If it ain't broke, don't fix it. But do change the oil.

I could be wrong, but I really don't think I am. Whether it takes 20, 40, or 100 years, scientific orthodoxy will eventually catch up to the common sense of my telomere stem cell theory of aging and disease.

WHY WE AGE—REDUX

What is the unspeakable heresy of this book? We propose that when it comes to aging and the diseases associated with it, there is just one cause, which your body is designed to resist. This remedy, namely stem cell maintenance via telomerase activation in stem cells, is mediated through the six areas that we explored. If there is literally just one major process that results in all illness, decline, and aging, then that should be welcomed as good news. That isn't to say there aren't exceptions, because environmental factors such as infections do play a role; but an intact adaptive immune system is our trump card. And that isn't to say that there aren't rare genetic diseases that can arise in our gene pool. They can. But in general, most viable humans are sufficiently interbred so as to be free from serious inherited genetic diseases.

When most people say "genes," they are usually referring to some predetermined, inherited blessing or curse, but you now know that is wrong. Most diseases, handicaps, special abilities, characteristics, and/or endowments are mere potentialities that require one or two defective alleles in stem cells, as you learned in Chapter 2.

You also now understand that all your cells carry all your chromosomes, and that all the genes contained in your chromosomes are potentially damaged by replicative senescence. Remember, telomere shortening from copying without adequate telomerase replacement leads to chromothripsis "chromosome confetti," which almost always leads to your cells melting themselves like little bad witches. We now view aging as a gradual mosaic accumulation of damaged versions of our cells that survive with damaged genes; after we acquire enough mutations at a cellular level, we observe disease and dysfunction at the organ level.

Aging is an emergent property of processes best described by comparing it to three Hindu deities: Brahma the creator (stem cells), Vishnu the preserver (telomerase), and Shiva the destroyer (natural cell death). When there is an imbalance or deficiency of any of the trimurti (Hindu for "three forms"), you have illness and aging.

Let's say that Brahma, represented by the immortal stem cells, is damaged; you would have the chimerism or mosaicism of old age. Aging is the depletion of your mesenchymal stem cell reserves and the inevitable genetic drift away from pristine genomic integrity. Instead of one version of genes when you were a one-celled zygote, you cannot help but acquire deviant versions of your genetic code in stem cell lines simply from the inherent rate of typographical errors to say nothing of the rapid crescendo enabled by telomere attrition and chromosome breaks. A loss in the quality of stem cells is at the heart of the "Redenbacher effect," of getting a crescendo of diseases in your 70s because all the potential immortal replacement mesenchymal stem cells are now damaged goods.

In a promising study stem cell scientists took mesenchymal stem cells, replicated them *in vitro*, then reintroduced them into osteoporotic mice to reverse their disease. There is no reason why such an approach wouldn't work in humans as long as we can isolate those good copies and make sure damaged ones can be coaxed into early retirement.

Vishnu is the preserver and represents telomerase activation. At the risk of confusing you, what if I told you that telomerase activation is not only the cure for aging, but also a big part of the problem? Much of the aging phenotype comes from cells that have overstayed their welcome and acquired too many mutations from any number of sources, such as copying but also environmental mutagens? Yes, the telomerase slows them from mutating at the natural pace, but it can also keep the older and damaged chromosomes from shortening to the point of chromothripsis (diffuse chromosomal entropy) that triggers p53 activation and desirable cell suicide. There is another accomplice in stem cell maintenance, called FOXO4 protein, which we will discuss in the next section.

Since immortality is "always on" in stem cells, we tend to accumulate more ornery and dysfunctional stem cells as we age. This failure to suicide is relatively common as shown by a study revealing how loss-of-heterozygosity p53 mutations occur in stem cell lines. Not surprisingly, this study showed that cells that lost the ability to kill themselves, but retained immortality conferred by telomerase activity, tended to not kill themselves but to stick around, causing problems such as cancer, at a high rate.

Thankfully, this is where the third Hindu deity, Shiva the destroyer, represented by cellular death, steps in. Most people view destruction as a negative thing, but without death there would be no renewal. Luckily, there are processes like exercised-induced destruction and radiation in low doses to help cells mutate and die. The misunderstood truth is that cancer treatments of chemo and radiation, when they are successful, accelerate genetic damage and cause hyper-aging in cancer cells (along with all the collateral damage of non-cancer healthy regular and stem cells). But this still requires the same intact suicide pathways. Studies in mice show that if we help to reduce the inhibition p53-mediated suicide of damaged cells, the organism can be restored to a more youthful state. Think of FOXO4 as a dampener on p53. By making a molecule that looks like this dampener but doesn't act like it, you have a classic competitive inhibitor and this unbridles p53 to cause cell death.

As we learned in Chapter 2, chromosomal mutation from telomere shortening, end-to-end fusion, and non-dysfunction is meant to trigger cell suicide by p53-mediated self-immolation via popping the mitochondria piñatas filled with battery acid. Yes, cell death can also be externally imposed as per cytotoxic T lymphocytes that hunt down virally infected or cancerous cells, but each cell, as a "prime directive" if you will, has many mechanisms to detect problems and multiple ways to kill itself off. None are more important than p53, although there are other ways to activate Lord Shiva from within.

So in summation, aging is an emergent property of three Hindu deities. You have telomerase immortalizing (Vishnu) the damaged but eternally copying stem cells (Brahma) that are not bad enough to kill themselves off yet (Shiva). The accumulation of not-so-good but not-so-bad stem cells is like having the Greek Olympic team from fifty years ago still representing the country fifty years later due to union rules. It may be logical and serve some purpose, but it isn't the best team you could be fielding, and is likely creating a clubhouse environment that is cranky, in pain, and going to get hurt.

HOW TO GET TO EXTRA INNINGS

In American baseball, the game is scheduled to last just nine innings, or eight and a half, depending on who is winning. There is no such thing as a tie in baseball, so that is why, at the end of each inning, if the score is tied, the game is extended into extra innings. Let's say an inning equals a decade of your life, and your "game" is currently designed to go from eight and a half to nine innings. What if you could tweak your trimurti to achieve what Wade Boggs, Cal Ripken, Jr., and Bob Ojeda achieved when the Pawtucket Red Sox went 32 innings with the Rochester Red Wings in an April 18, 1981, Triple A game? Would you want to live 320 years? Is it possible? At some point in the not too distant future, science will get better at destroying damaged stem cells, extracting and analyzing existing stem cells, and then replenishing them for clinical use. Once they do that, we have a pretty good shot at living healthier and longer lives. None of these technologies is far-fetched—it will just take a little time and will to actualize them within our lifetimes. In the meantime, your job is to preserve the best copies of your stem cells you can.

What are some of the keys to staying alive until practical stem cell therapy is available? Live mindfully with the six TMT cylinders and focus on the other six cylinders of enjoyment, presence, authenticity, productivity, gratitude, and self-compassion. Don't get caught up in the latest health fads. The very nature of intellectual property monetization via drug development means that no one is going to actively promote an effective cure for aging. Why would a multi-billion dollar company seek to put all their other business divisions out of operation?

Moderation is key, although people don't find that appealing. The U-shaped curve of exercise benefit can also apply to body fat percentage, and probably many other things such as time spent at home, thoughts about the future, vacations taken, and so on. The middle pathway may not seem like the sexiest, but it is often the most prudent.

Everything old is new again. Laughter IS the best medicine and there is laughter yoga, laughter therapy, and let's face it, there is a lot to laugh at if you are being honest. I had the pleasure of meeting and treating a 114-year-old woman and what I most clearly remember was that she never stopped trying to crack a joke.

Finally, this book is your ally and resource as well. Rather than subject you to some checklist of dos and don'ts, I've tried to give you the tools to interpret science and personal experience in a way that would best serve you. What makes you happy in terms of exercise and diet is ultimately unique and personal. You can't really *hurt* yourself that easily, as the cylinders are always working on your behalf; but there are plenty of ways to optimize once you learn the fundamentals and how to monitor and adjust how you are living.

There was a movie based on a true story called *Into the Wild*, where an alienated young man went to escape into the Alaskan wilderness only to starve and die alone. The irony was that less than a mile away, there was a hand-operated tram that he could have used to cross the river back to safety. Perhaps escaping the aging process is also much well within your reach.[1]

THE TRANSHUMAN QUESTION

The major crossroads that faces man is the question of transhumanism. The benefits of transhumanism, which can be interpreted as improvements to the human form via incorporating technologies, are significant. We already use glasses and refractive surgery to improve vision, insulin pumps to manage insulin, and artificial organs and limbs to some extent.

Some powerful transhuman technologies will be the ability to edit genetic code and operate on chromosomes, the invention of new types of organelles and symbiotic microbes, and even the production of free-roaming nanocytes, or robotic policemen that can carry out certain functions on behalf of your doctor. Gene editing has long been possible but is now being popularized by the CRISPR/Cas9 system. The ability to add extra copies of telomerase via gene therapy is a technology that has existed since 1989 but was only tried as recently as 2015. In general, I believe that such technologies are misguided attempts to solve the wrong problem. We carry around with us perfectly good copies of our genome that can be sequenced and archived in our 20s. For most of our adult lives, we carry around with us mesenchymal stem cells of high genomic integrity that can be repurposed. And we are starting to learn what signaling molecules naturally enhance youthful behaviors of stem cells.

The ability of artificial technology to interact with human neural circuitry is advancing at a rapid pace, much to the delight of some and chagrin of others. What will the 24-hour monitoring and uploading and downloading of information to an all-knowing cloud authority mean for the human condition with regard to privacy and freedom?

If I had to answer whether transhumanism would prove to be a blessing or a curse, I would say that it would mostly be bad news. I am philosophically resistant to any technology that doesn't work with existing biology but instead invites new problems and unforeseen consequences in the name of unbridled progress. Since the human soul is not undergoing as rapid an evolution as our technology, the morally challenged among us, who already disproportionally tend to control the companies and agencies that will deploy this technology, might view transhumanism as an opportunity for profit and influence rather than a betterment of the species.

The human machine as it currently exists is simply a few minor tweaks away from being effectively immortal. The ability to read and influence minds across the planet or shoot lasers from our fingertips would seem to me little to elevate the human spirit and inviting always-on cognitive interfacing, nano-machines, engineered bacteria, and genetic mutation seems to be the prelude to a sci-fi horror story that we don't want to see played out.

THE FUTURE IS BOUNDLESS AND, HOPEFULLY, HUMAN

So it must be said that we live in a world that is not as it is but rather as we believe. If we improve our personal beliefs, we improve the quality of our lives. If we believe in a future that is more abundant and just, then we help to create such a world.

If we wish to live in the Dark Ages again, we can choose to believe what some serious experts believe, and accept with religious fervor that scarcity of resources and scarcity of years are preordained.

Alternatively, you can embrace the scientific method and learn from the many examples of natural and artificial engineering or immortality. As for this moment in time, we must look to the ancient wisdom to make sense of the current telomere science. There is only one disease and everything is an interconnected system. Your happy thoughts influence your happy cells, and help to regrow happy and healthy telomeres. Even if you don't go in for all that New Age spiritualism, yoga, meditation, and Mediterranean diets, just realize that you probably only have to put up with it for a decade or two before extreme longevity will be scientifically available.

Would you want to live 320 years? Probably not. However, what if you and all your loved ones could maintain the body and functioning of a 21-year-old? You just might be willing to give that a go, I'll bet. By then, you could be a poet, a musician, an actor and playwright, or maybe a champion in several sports. You might hop a transport to another part of the world to decide to learn a new language—just don't let them implant a chip for that purpose, because we already create enough demons and malware programs in our minds without actually needing them installed. I truly believe that most of us were endowed with a high-functioning, nearly flawless machinery and that we just need to keep it well oiled until we can learn to reliably replace damaged stem cells in a sustainable fashion.

Perhaps you worry that you would get so bored with yourself that you would want to die just to feel some change? Doubtful, unless you had a way to transfer your consciousness in a reliable way to another form or dimension. As Hamlet said, "Thus conscience [meaning consciousness] does make cowards of us all."[2] In other words, if we knew for certain what fate was awaiting us in the afterlife (the undiscovered country), we might just opt out of this one's "slings and arrows of outrageous fortune."

I hope you have enjoyed our wild excursion through my theories, your physiology, and your personal wellness plans. I look forward to hearing your feedback about how this new understanding and self-assessment technology has changed your paradigms of health and wellness and enriched the lives of those around you as well. Don't forget that to serve is why we are here. Be of service to yourself first, but then share that joy and compassion with the world in a scalable, fractal, expansive pattern of even more resonance and joy.

So here's to occasionally rereading this book and to sticking to your TeloMirror self-assessments nightly or just from time to time. Stay grateful. Breath consciously. C.A.R.E. when you are anxious, and sleep more than you think is morally acceptable. Be skeptical of advice that labels anything you find pleasurable as absolutely good or bad. You should never expect to be perfect, happy, contented, or immortal; but you should never stop trying either, for those aspirations are what make the journey so meaningful and satisfying.

Thank you for your patience, attention, willingness to suspend disbelief, and for your hard work. I hope this book helped you to believe in an alternative reality where you don't have to get sicker and older, where abundance and wellness are a given, and that it didn't amount to so much "sound and fury" from a mind that spends too much time dreaming while awake.

POSTSCRIPT

In case you missed them, here are the 12 epigraphs I wrote for each chapter. I think they pretty well sum up this journey we have taken together:

Chapter 1: The Quest to End Aging

*Question all you believe and
believe only what you've questioned.*

Chapter 2: Biology 101—Genetics and Cell Biology

Truth is easy to grasp and hard to vary.

Chapter 3: Aging—One Cause, One Cure

Intuition is the royal road to wisdom.

Chapter 4: Your Breath

Breathe in, breathe out. Repeat until death.

Chapter 5: Your Mind

Seeing isn't believing. It works the other way around.

Chapter 6: Your Sleep

*Today seemed a regrettable
and pointless interruption of sleep.*

Chapter 7: Your Exercise

*The heart is made of muscle. Muscles grow
stronger with use and can't be broken.*

Chapter 8: Your Diet

*"We must eat fruits and vegetables to live."
— No Eskimo, ever*

Chapter 9: Your Supplements

*Step right up, son. I hold in my
hand the ancient elixir of eternal life!*

Chapter 10: What Do You See in Your TeloMirrors?

The only thing that makes sense is change.

Chapter 11: Your TeloMirror Tune-Up

I'm so happy now I can barely stand myself.

Chapter 12: The Future Is Ageless

If it ain't broke, don't fix it. But do change the oil.

GLOSSARY

2-Arachidonoylglycerol (2-AG). An abundant endogenous (as opposed to plant-derived) signaling molecule that your body produces to interact with endocannabinoid receptors. Its levels are boosted by the use of cannabidiol (CBD), and it appears to play a significant role in immune modulation.

adaptogen. A substance, usually herbally derived, that has paradoxical and rebalancing effects upon physiology. A hallmark of an adaptogenic substance is that it will have different effects upon different people, such as making a sleep-deprived person sleep more and a hypersomnolent person sleep less.

antidiuretic hormone (ADH). A short-acting hormone produced by the hypothalamus and released by the posterior pituitary gland in response to low blood volume or high serum osmolality (thick blood associated with dehydration). ADH serves to prevent fluid loss, retain sodium, and constrict blood vessels. Inappropriate secretion can be caused by stress, pain, and drug reactions.

Attention Deficit Hyperactivity Disorder (ADHD). A syndrome characterized by problems paying attention, excessive activity, or difficulty controlling behavior.

adiponectin. A hormone produced by fat cells that is associated with body fat storage homeostasis. When it is deficient, it can be associated with obesity and insulin resistance (type 2 diabetes).

allele. Any variant of a gene that encodes a protein via transcription into messenger RNA. Although there are infinite numbers of alleles possible, in practice they are usually limited in the population due to common genetic ancestry and natural selection for functional alleles as a result of evolution.

alopecia. A general term meaning loss of hair.

alpha waves. The type of brain EEG activity seen when eyes are closed or during NREM1 (light sleep). Alpha brain wave activity is 8 to 12 cycles per second.

Alzheimer's disease. A serious and sometimes progressive loss of cognitive and neurological function often associated with advanced age. Alzheimer's is a poorly understood, multifactorial, and ill-defined disease that may have many contributing factors, including poor sleep and glymphatic drainage as well as gene mutations that confer a higher risk of manifesting the disease.

Ambien. Brand name for zolpidem, a commonly used and powerful sleep-inducing agent that can be associated with drug tolerance, dependence, and rebound insomnia. Brain waves while taking Ambien are lower in voltage, and therefore sleep is not normal in architecture or in restorative capacity.

amino acids. Building blocks of proteins that come in about 20 types in humans. These individual molecules are assembled using messenger RNA (mRNA) and gene translation into discrete proteins. Transfer RNA (tRNA) molecules are specialized to carry distinct amino acids and match them to the mRNA 3-nucleotide codon, depending on their tRNA matching 3-nucleotide anticodon sequence.

amphiphilic. Term describing a molecule that possesses both water solubility (hydrophilic) and fat solubility (hydrophobic) qualities. Soaps, bile salts, and phospholipids that make up cell membranes are all examples of amphiphilic molecules.

ampulla of Vater. A small projection into the duodenum, formed by the union of the pancreatic duct and the common bile duct; the site where the bile from the liver and the pancreatic digestive enzymes and bicarbonate enter the duodenum.

amylase. A digestive enzyme found in saliva and pancreatic fluid that breaks down complex sugars into simpler forms for absorption by the gastrointestinal tract.

anandamide. An endogenous fatty acid neurotransmitter whose name is derived from the Sanskrit word *ananda*, or "bliss." It activates both the CB1 and CB2 endocannabinoid receptors and generally improves mood. Various healthy lifestyle and mind-set changes may help to increase endogenous anandamide production (see *endocannabinoid*).

androgens. A class of 19-carbon steroid sex hormones that are associated with male reproductive function as well as secondary sex characteristics such as facial and body hair growth, sebaceous secretions, increased muscle mass, lower body fat, and voice deepening. Androgens are defined by their actions on androgen receptors and are made in the adrenal gland as well as the testes. Their decline in advanced age is known as andropause.

andropause. In contrast to female menopause, which has a clear etiology in cessation of ovulation, andropause is a theoretical and general descriptor for the signs and symptoms associated with declining male hormone levels that can occur with advanced age.

aneuploid. Having an improper number of chromosomes. In a typical human, there are 46 chromosomes. Any number more or less than this is considered aneuploid. The major driver of aneuploidy is breakage and uneven segregation made possible by fused chromosomes created by DNA double strand breakage repair after telomere erosion.

antioxidants. Electron-donating molecules that inhibit loss of electrons (oxidation), which can cause free radical, reactive oxygen species (ROS), and biochemical damage. Natural antioxidants include glutathione and vitamin C.

antisense strand. The $3' \rightarrow 5'$ (read as "three prime to five prime"), leading, negative, or antisense strand is the half of DNA that reads the opposite of the mRNA transcript ($5' \rightarrow 3'$). It is used to transcribe the mRNA (see *mRNA*, *leading strand*, and *mRNA or gene translation*).

apoptosis. Intentional cell suicide caused by either an external call for assassination by the immune system or an internal triggering of mitochondrial lysis. A major trigger for programmed cell death is aneuploidy, brought about by telomere erosion and end-to-end fusion, which is detected by p53, the "watchman of the genome."

Asperger's syndrome. A relatively milder form of autism in which a person displays repetitive behaviors and interests while functioning poorly in nonverbal communication and social interaction (see *autism*).

astragalus (huang qi). A genus of plants that contains some substances long used in Traditional Chinese Medicine to enhance longevity, immunity, and qi (life force). Extracts of astragalus have been used as telomerase activators, such as TA-65.

asymmetric division. Division of one cell into two dissimilar copies: one is a perfect copy of a stem mother and the other is a more differentiated daughter.

asthma. An inflammatory condition resulting in muscular spasms of the airways. This produces difficulty breathing as well as wheezing, coughing, and shortness of breath. Triggers for asthma are generally allergic but can also include exercise and cold air.

adenosine triphosphate (ATP). A nucleotide made up of a nucleic acid (adenine), a sugar (ribose), and three linked phosphates. It can be less "charged" if it contains only one phosphate (adenosine monophosphate, or AMP) or two phosphates (adenosine diphosphate, or ADP). The process of making ATP in oxidative phosphorylation creates the universal currency for powering the body (see *cellular respiration*).

ATP synthase. The enzyme embedded in the inner membrane of the mitochondria that uses the electrical gradient of protons generated by the electron transport train to generate ATP, the universal currency of biochemistry (see *adenosine triphosphate* and *oxidative phosphorylation*).

autism. A mental condition characterized by unusual and age-inappropriate difficulty with language, relationships, social interactions, and nonverbal communication (see *Asperger's syndrome* and *theory of mind*).

autonomic nervous system. The unconscious control system for bodily functions such as heart rate, digestion, respiratory rate, pupillary response, urination, and sexual arousal. It has two main opposing yet cooperative divisions: the excitatory sympathetic nervous system (fight or flight) and the relaxing parasympathetic nervous system (restore and relax).

autophagy. The "self-eating" mechanisms by which a cell takes unused or dysfunctional materials, digests them, and extrudes them. It involves surrounding the unwanted substances with a spherical membrane, then fusing it to a destructive lysosome, then extruding the waste. Autophagy is a normal, healthy process and is encouraged by periods of fasting.

autosomal dominant. Refers to a pattern of Mendelian genetic inheritance in which a disease condition will manifest when even one healthy or wild type allele is present. An example of an autosomal dominant disease is accelerated aging, or progeria, from dyskeratosis congenita, a condition where one of the alleles involved in telomerase activity is abnormal.

autosomal recessive. Refers to a pattern of Mendelian genetic inheritance whereby having one non-wild type or defective allele will not generally manifest as a disease state unless loss of heterozygosity occurs in a stem cell line. In contrast, autosomal dominant diseases can manifest without the full gene dosage of wild type inheritance from both maternal and paternal genomes (see *gene dosage*).

axons. The relatively long appendage of a neuron that transmits electrical impulses to a receiving and possibly relaying nerve cell (the postsynaptic neuron). Axons require myelin to efficiently conduct electricity (see *myelin*).

base pair. A unit consisting of two matching nucleotides bound to each other by hydrogen bonds. Base pairs form the building blocks of the DNA double helix like rungs on a ladder. A base pair is also used as the unit of measure for DNA molecule length.

beriberi. Condition caused by vitamin B1 (thiamine) nutritional deficiency. Symptoms include severe neurological and psychological problems such as sensory difficulties, weakness, poor balance, confusion, and psychosis. First recognized when fixed diets consisting of polished rice were common; populations such as prisoners or refugees with limited food variety and no vitamin fortification are at risk.

beta-amyloid. A brain protein of unclear function that can accumulate into plaques in Alzheimer's disease. Beta-amyloid is cleared by the glymphatic system during sleep (see *glymphatic system*).

beta brain waves. The measured normal brain activity of relatively low amplitude and high frequency between 12 and 38 cycles per second that occurs during waking consciousness with eyes open. When eyes are closed or while dreaming in REM sleep, the brain displays higher amplitude, lower frequency (8 to 12 cycles per second) alpha waves (see *alpha waves* and *REM sleep*).

bile salts (bile acids). Amphiphilic molecules made in the liver, stored in the gallbladder, and released into the duodenum that serve to emulsify and package digested fats and fat-soluble vitamins (A, D, E, K) for absorption in the ileum.

bilirubin. A yellow breakdown product of hemoglobin that is excreted into the bile. When the liver is damaged, increased blood levels of bilirubin show up as yellow skin and eyes, or jaundice. After breakdown by gut bacteria, bilirubin metabolites are what make urine appear yellow (urobilin) and stool brown (stercobilin).

Brahma. In Hinduism, the god of creation, forming one part of the *trimurti* (three forms) along with Vishnu the preserver and Shiva the destroyer. Although responsible for creating the physical world, Brahma is said to be dependent on a higher metaphysical reality and therefore is often depicted as arising from a lotus growing from the navel of Vishnu.

BRCA1/BRCA2. Oncogenes responsible for higher rates of cancer when defective. Both genes are involved in double strand breakage repair and, when affected by point mutations, can confer disease if both wild type genes are affected or loss of heterozygosity occurs (see *double strand breakage repair*, *point mutation*, and *loss of heterozygyosity*).

C-reactive protein. A nonspecific marker of inflammation produced by the liver in response to immune activity. Its role is to coat dying cells and pathogens in order to activate the complement system, a cascade of biological chemical reactions that attract more immune cells, invite those cells to consume damaged cells and pathogens, and help to destroy cell walls of complement-coated cells and pathogens.

C.A.R.E. A mnemonic created by the author to explain a meditative technique for managing a busy mind. The steps are Clearing, Auditing, Reframing, and Enjoying.

carbon dioxide. Carbon dioxide is produced by aerobic cellular respiration. Oxygen and glucose are used by cells to create ATP, water, heat, and CO_2 as by-products (see *cellular respiration*).

computerized axial tomography (CAT scan). A computer-assisted imaging technology that uses multiple X-rays from different angles to assemble virtual "slices" around an axis. This technology involves substantially more potentially DNA-damaging radiation exposure than simple X-rays or MRI (see *MRI*).

cannabidiol (CBD). One of the active molecules in cannabis that doesn't produce psychotropic changes. It acts as an indirect antagonist of both CB1 and CB2 receptors, possibly causing upregulation of those receptors and potentiating the effects of tetrahydrocannabinol (THC). CBD also may inhibit anandamide reuptake and breakdown and thereby act as a natural antianxiety compound, similar to pharmacological serotonin reuptake inhibitors (SSRIs).

cellular respiration. Metabolic reactions that occur in the cell and its mitochondria that serve to convert nutritional molecules into ATP, the universal currency for energy-requiring reactions. The process in animals requires oxygen to power a process called oxidative phosphorylation via the electron transport chain (see *Krebs cycle*, *oxidative phosphorylation*, and *electron transport chain*).

cholecystokinin. A hormone released by the mucosal cells lining the duodenum and jejunum in response to the presence of food and need for digestive assistance. It delays stomach emptying (allowing for chemical digestion to take place) and stimulates the release of bile and pancreatic fluids such as bicarbonate and digestive enzymes of amylase, protease, and lipase.

chromosome. A discrete DNA molecule used by eukaryotic (nucleus-having) cells to store genetic information. The chromosomes of two "daughter" cells are inherited from one "mother" cell (or two gametes, in the case of a fertilized egg) and consist of double-stranded DNA sometimes wrapped around histones (proteins that act like spools).

chromothripsis. A general term for significant disorder and rearrangements in chromosomal number and internal ordering. Several causes have been proposed for chromothripsis, including micronuclei formation (genetic division that occurs apart from the main chromosomal contingent), aborted apoptosis, and end-to-end fusion from telomere dysfunction (see *apoptosis* and *end-to-end fusion*).

cilia. In the context of lung function, cilia are slender projections from cells lining the respiratory tract that sweep mucus up and out of the lungs, as if sweeping ashes back up a chimney. These cilia work together in coordinated waves and create phlegm.

cytomegalovirus (CMV). Cytomegalovirus is a very prevalent chronic virus that causes lifelong infection in humans. As with many of the herpesvirus family viruses, it is impossible to eradicate. CMV may also play a central role in the exhaustion of the immune system and therefore in aging itself.

complementary strand. The precisely paired DNA strand that matches another strand.

chronic obstructive pulmonary disease (COPD). A category of progressive conditions resulting from different causes but ultimately producing poor air flow in the lungs. Shortness of breath, chronic cough, wheezing, and performance on lung function tests can help distinguish the most common two forms of COPD: chronic bronchitis and emphysema.

CoQ10. A molecule present in the mitochondria that is an active participant in the electron transport chain reactions that enable oxidative phosphorylation (see *cellular respiration* and *oxidative phosphorylation*).

cortisol. A hormone produced by the adrenal gland in response to stress or low blood glucose. It triggers increased blood sugar and suppresses the immune system.

Continuous Positive Airway Pressure (CPAP). A respiratory assisting technological device that blows air (hopefully heated and humidified) into the airways of the sleeper in order to prevent the airway collapse that occurs with obstructive sleep apnea (see *sleep apnea*).

central processing unit (CPU). In computing, the CPU is where the "thinking" of the computer takes place.

crankshaft. A mechanical engine part that translates the up-and-down force of pistons into a rotational motion or vice versa.

Crohn's disease. An inflammatory disease of unknown origin that mainly affects the gastrointestinal tract, characterized by abdominal pain, diarrhea, fever, and weight loss. It produces ulcers, fistulas (erosive communication between noncontiguous viscera), and blockages or obstructions.

Ctrl-Alt-Delete. The simultaneous pressing of these three buttons can call up the Task Manager in a Windows-based computer. The Task Manager displays some of the current active processes, programs, and performance that are occurring and affecting your computer's CPU and memory.

cystic fibrosis. A relatively common autosomal-recessive genetic disease caused by two nonfunctioning alleles of the cystic fibrosis transmembrane conductance gene. Its name derives from the fibrosis and cysts formed in the pancreas. The disease causes problems in the lungs, liver, intestines, and kidneys.

declarative memory. Also known as explicit memory. Specific facts, events, or details that can be recalled, such as phone numbers, word definitions, faces, and sense memories. Declarative memory is made during slow wave sleep, in contrast to procedural memory, which is attended to during REM sleep (see *slow wave sleep, procedural memory,* and *REM sleep*).

delta brain waves. In deepest NREM3, or slow wave sleep, delta brain waves of high amplitude and low frequency (0.5 to 3 cycles per second) dominate. During this deep and restorative sleep, some sleep spindles occur, but the state of consciousness is generally dreamless and the sleeper is paralyzed and unaware of his or her surroundings (see NREM3).

differentiated cells. An abstract concept implying more cellular specialization and less potentiality of stemness. Cell differentiation occurs not on the genetic level but primarily on the epigenetic level by virtue of gene expression modulation governed by RNA and other chemical modifications (see *stemness* and *epigenetic*).

deoxyribonucleic acid (DNA). Molecules that come in four types and assemble into polymer chains, which then pair by specific rules to a complementary strand in order to form a double helix. DNA is the common information storage medium for all life on Earth, except a few certain RNA viruses, and is inherited between generations of cells as well as organisms (see *complementary strand*).

double strand breakage repair. A system of DNA surveillance and repair by proteins that finds and splices breaks in chromosomal continuity such as might occur from ionizing radiation. When this system detects discontinuity, it reconnects broken double-stranded DNA. In the context of telomere erosion, an uncapped or critically short chromosomal end will be recognized by the double strand breakage repair system and inappropriately joined to another chromosome, if possible, resulting in end-to-end fusion, aneuploidy, and usually apoptosis (see *end-to-end fusion*).

Dunning-Kruger effect. A psychological term named for the scientists who described the cognitive bias of people with low ability to overestimate their competence owing to their deficiency of metacognition (thinking about thinking). A corollary of the Dunning-Kruger effect is that people of higher competence mistakenly assume that others can function at their level of cognition.

duodenum. The segment of small intestine between the stomach and jejunum that receives the fluids from the pancreas, liver, and gallbladder. The ampulla of Vater is the spigot through which those fluids pass into the canal or lumen of the duodenum.

dyskeratosis congenita. A disease of accelerated aging manifesting mainly as abnormal skin, lung fibrosis, and early bone marrow failure in the presence of accelerated telomere shortening. Many of the autosomal dominant forms of this inherited disease involve mutations in alleles or genes involved in the telomerase system and result from a less than full gene dosage.

electroencephalogram (EEG). An indirect method of measuring brain activity by placing electrodes over the brain (usually on the scalp). During different types of mental activity and states of consciousness, various patterns of activity are measured (see *alpha waves, beta waves, delta waves, theta waves,* and *gamma waves*).

electron transport chain. A series of proteins bound to the inner membrane of the mitochondria that transfer electrons from electron donors to electron acceptors via REDOX reactions. This enables an electrical gradient of protons to be created and the flow of those protons back across the membrane powers ATP synthase, the enzyme that produces ATP (see *oxidative phosphorylation, NADH,* and *CoQ10*).

end-replication problem. A concept for the mechanical impossibility of copying linear DNA to the very end (see *lagging strand* and *Okazaki fragments*).

end-to-end fusion. Fusion of previously distinct chromosomes that is enabled by telomere erosion and double strand DNA breakage repair. This irreversible process leads to both breakage and uneven chromosomal segregation between daughter cells (aneuploidy) after cell division. When p53, the "watchman of the genome," detects an improper chromosomal number, it can initiate cell suicide, or apoptosis.

endocannabinoid. Pertaining to a system of neuromodulatory receptors that interact with endogenous signals (such as anandamide or 2-AG) or their cannabis-derived analogues (THC and CBD). Activities that increase relaxation tend to increase endocannabinoids and thereby promote efficient cellular functioning.

entropy. The concept of disintegration of order or predictability.

enzyme. A protein produced in cells by assembling amino acids in a process known as mRNA translation. Enzymes are catalysts and often specialized "machines" that perform tasks needed for biochemical and physiological reactions. The chemical composition and ways in which proteins fold determine the enzymes' function (see *amino acids* and *mRNA or gene translation*).

epigenetic. Meaning "outside the genes," this is an imprecise and broad term to describe inheritable traits in cells that are not attributable to the simple genetic code of the chromosomal DNA. It can include RNA modifications, chemical modification such as acetylation and methylation, and even organelles.

esophagus. A fibromuscular, peristaltic tube that connects the mouth to the stomach. It has a sphincter to prevent reflux of stomach acid backward, but when that fails, "heartburn" can occur.

essential amino acids. The 9 out of 20 amino acids that cannot be synthesized in the human body and therefore must be ingested in the diet.

essential fatty acids. Fatty acids that cannot be synthesized by the human body and must therefore be ingested. The two known types are omega-3 and omega-6 fatty acids.

estrogens. A class of steroid sex hormone associated with female reproduction and secondary sex characteristics such as breast enlargement, wide hips, fat distribution around buttocks and thighs, round face, and softer features. The precipitous loss of estrogens due to menopause accelerates aging in women, as the fat cells, liver, adrenal glands, and breasts cannot make up for this loss.

fatigued athlete myopathic syndrome (FAMS). A disorder of muscle structure and function associated with overuse. There is a correlation between short telomeres in the muscle stem cells and this condition.

fast-twitch muscles. A type of muscle fiber specialized for short bursts, such as lifting heavy weights or sprinting, which can operate under conditions without oxygen. These fast-twitch muscles are harder to maintain in advanced age.

fat-soluble vitamins. Vitamins A, D, E, and K are fat soluble and therefore require bile acids to be absorbed. Vitamin D can also be synthesized with exposure to sunlight and vitamin K can be synthesized by gut bacteria.

fatal familial insomnia. A rare disease resulting from knockout of the ability to form prions, which enable normal sleep and memory formation. Sufferers are unable to enter deeper sleep beyond stage NREM1 and will die within 18 months, essentially from the secondary effects of sleep deprivation.

fecal transplantation. The process of transferring stool from the colon of a healthy person to one harboring pathogenic bacteria with the hope of obtaining a probiotic result. With the exception of antibiotic-induced *Clostridium difficile* infection, fecal transplantation is of unproven benefit, given the high counts of diverse and relatively benign enteric bacteria that inhabit the colon and make up as much as 50 percent of the biomass of stool (see *probiotic*).

functional MRI (fMRI). A form of dynamic magnetic-resonance imaging that infers where functional brain activity is occurring in real time for the purposes of mapping out thought processes. Oxygenated hemoglobin looks different in this imaging, and so in areas where there is higher oxygen delivery, it is inferred that those neurons are most active.

FOXO4. A protein that naturally inhibits the apoptotic action of p53 and thereby delays self-destruction of senescent and genetically damaged cells. Inhibition of FOXO4 accelerates senolysis, or destruction of old cells (see *p53* and *apoptosis*).

fused chromosomes. Joining together of previously separate chromosomes. In the context of evolution, previous discrete chromosomes fused to become joined in distinct species. In the context of replicative senescence that occurs in all dividing cells, when telomeres shorten excessively, the DNA double strand breakage repair inappropriately treats these uncapped ends as breaks and joins them to other chromosomes, resulting in end-to-end fusions.

GABA. The chief inhibitory neurotransmitter of the brain. When GABA is present, the brain is able to relax. When it is suppressed—for example, by the excess of glutamine produced hours after alcohol consumption—the brain is more wakeful and less able to benefit from the regenerative properties of sleep (see *glutamine*).

gamma waves. High-frequency brain waves of 38 or greater cycles per second that may occur with high levels of perception, focus, and compassion. Advanced practitioners of meditation can generate this brain wave pattern when thinking about compassion.

gene dosage. Refers to the number of copies of an allele, usually the healthy and common wild type. Although examples can occur with greater than two copies and hence a higher than binary gene dosage, typically the number is zero (double knockout), one (heterozygous), or two (homozygous, with both parents contributing a healthy gene allele via Mendelian genetic inheritance).

gene transcription. The transfer of a discrete gene sequence, composed of antisense DNA, to a complementary sense (5'→3') messenger RNA (mRNA). This mRNA gene transcript will travel out of the nucleus to be used in mRNA or gene translation in the cytoplasm by ribosomes.

genes. A specific gene is a heritable sequence of coding DNA that specifies the discrete mRNA (see mRNA) transcript for a specific sequence of amino acids that will be assembled into a protein by mRNA translation. In general, sexually reproducing organisms receive a maternal and paternal copy of most genes in a process known as Mendelian Genetics (see *allele, mRNA or gene translation,* and *Mendelian genetics*).

genome. A cell's complete set of genetic information. In eukaryotic cells, the genome consists of the chromosomes housed in the cellular nucleus.

glucagon. Produced by the pancreas in response to low blood sugar levels. It triggers the breakdown of fats and carbohydrates and the synthesis of new glucose. Glucagon works in opposition to another pancreatic hormone, insulin, which lowers blood glucose by transporting it into cells for fat storage (see *gluconeogenesis*).

gluconeogenesis. The formation of glucose by breakdown of glycogen or synthesis from amino acids or fat metabolites. In response to low blood sugar (hypoglycemia), gluconeogenesis is triggered.

glucose. A simple six-carbon sugar used as the primary exchange currency for energy; can be made from ingested fats, proteins, and sugars. Blood glucose levels are maintained in a narrow range by the opposing pancreatic hormones of insulin and glucagon.

glutamine. An amino acid that plays a positive role in wakefulness. Consumption of alcohol before sleep temporarily suppresses glutamine production; in response, the body produces an excess of glutamine, which results in GABA suppression, inability to sleep deeply, wakefulness, and hangovers (see *GABA*).

glycemic index. A relative measure of the ability of ingested sugars to cause elevation in blood glucose and therefore trigger insulin release and fat storage. Glucose has a high glycemic index of 100 (or 100 percent). Sugars in processed foods, such as maltose and high fructose corn syrup, and white breads and polished rice have high glycemic indices, whereas sugars from natural plant sources have lower glycemic indices and are therefore less fattening.

glycolysis. The breakdown of six-carbon glucose, a simple sugar, into two three-carbon pyruvate molecules to power the citric acid cycle. In this process, two ATP and two NADH (a molecule that powers the electron transport chain) are also netted.

glymphatic system. A portmanteau word from *glial* (the support cells of the brain) and *lymphatic* (a system for circulating interstitial, or extracellular but nonvascular, fluid). The brain, especially during sleep, uses the glymphatic system to remove waste products by expansion and increased flow between cells, like a wet sponge being rinsed.

goiter. A physiologic enlargement of the thyroid gland. Historically, its most common cause was nutritional iodine deficiency in areas without marine sources of food prior to the addition of iodine to table salt. Low levels of thyroid hormone caused by iodine deficiency cause the hypothalamus and pituitary to secrete a hormone that causes the thyroid gland to enlarge.

GRAS (Generally Recognized as Safe). A designation under the federal Food, Drug, and Cosmetic Act that a substance is deemed by qualified experts to be safe when used as intended. GRAS substances are exempt from being considered food additives.

Hayflick limit. A conceptual and empirical limitation on the number of population doublings or cell divisions that can occur before telomere shortening renders that cell line nonviable, usually as the result of end-to-end fusion and aneuploidy from cell and DNA replication. The Hayflick limit is 40 to 60 doublings, although this will vary depending on the preexisting telomere lengths (see *replicative senescence*).

hepatitis A. A virus producing liver infection and inflammation that is transmitted by fecal-oral contamination of food or water. The infection, unlike hepatitis B and C, is usually self-limited and can be relatively asymptomatic.

homeostasis. The ability or tendency to maintain balance and consistency rather than becoming unstable. An example would be maintenance of the body temperature in a narrow healthy range by behaviors, shivering, and other heat generation and dissipation.

hypnogram. A graphical representation in time of the phases of sleep derived from EEG activity, serving to characterize sleep architecture. Sleep architecture is the way in which phases of sleep, such as NREM1, NREM2, NREM3, and REM sleep, occur in a person; and hypnograms show that earlier cycles are dominated by NREM2 and NREM3 whereas later cycles are dominated by REM and NREM2 sleep.

hypothalamus. A region of the brain that controls the autonomic nervous system and pituitary gland by monitoring blood hormones and neurological input. It controls body temperature, thirst, hunger, and many other systems.

ileocecal valve. The muscular sphincter that separates the relatively sterile small intestines from the heavily contaminated large intestines, or colon.

ilium. The final part of the small intestines after the jejunum and before the large intestine or colon. It is specialized for reabsorption of vitamin B12 and bile salts, which form micelles, or soapy bubbles that can transport fats and fat-soluble molecules into the bloodstream from the intestinal tract (see *vitamin B12* and *bile salts*).

insulin. A hormone produced by the pancreas in response to high blood sugar levels. It promotes transport of glucose into fat, liver, and muscle cells for storage as fat. Insulin works in opposition to another pancreatic hormone, glucagon, which triggers the breakdown of fats and carbohydrates and the synthesis of new glucose (see *gluconeogenesis*).

introception. With regard to cognition, introception is the gathering and processing of information pertaining to the state of our body, such as spatial position, pain, skin sensations, hunger, temperature, bladder control, etcetera.

idiopathic pulmonary fibrosis (IPF). Idiopathic pulmonary fibrosis (i.e., lung scarring of unknown cause) is a descriptive category of conditions rather than a discrete entity. There are forms of this condition that have been directly associated with mutations in the components of telomerase activation.

jejunum. The middle part of the small intestines, after the duodenum and before the ileum, that is specialized with high surface area villi, or fingerlike projections similar to shag carpet. It allows for the absorption of small molecules such as sugars, amino acids, and smaller fat molecules.

K-complexes. A specific, relatively low then high voltage burst of brain activity that occurs during NREM2 sleep and is often followed by sleep spindles. K-complexes may occur in response to stimuli but also occur fairly regularly and spontaneously, leading researchers to believe they play a role in declarative memory formation in NREM2 and NREM3 sleep.

ketogenic diet. A diet that is low in or devoid of carbohydrate intake triggers gluconeogenesis, which entails the breakdown of fat into molecules known as ketones that can be used to create the glucose needed to power cellular respiration.

ketosis. During times of low blood glucose, breakdown of fats as a result of gluconeogenesis triggered by glucagon causes accumulation of fat breakdown products known as ketones that can be used to make new glucose. This ketosis is the basis of efficient weight loss in certain carbohydrate-poor diets (see *lipolysis* and *ketogenic diet*).

Krebs cycle (aka citric acid cycle). A series of chemical reactions in oxygen-using organisms that ultimately convert food molecules into chemical energy in the form of ATP and NADH (which powers oxidative phosphorylation).

lagging strand. See *sense strand*.

low-density lipoprotein (LDL). Commonly known as "bad cholesterol" because of its association with atherosclerosis. Lipoproteins transport lipids (fats) around the body as spherical vesicles of fat surrounded by proteins and a phospholipid shell. LDL is larger than HDL or IDL (high- and intermediate-density lipoproteins).

leading strand. See *antisense strand*.

leptin. The "satiety" hormone produced by adipose cells that feed back to the hypothalamus and suppress hunger. It is opposed by ghrelin, the "hungry" hormone produced when the stomach is empty or unstretched. Consumption of frequent smaller meals with plenty of water suppresses hunger by reducing stomach ghrelin production.

lipase. A digestive enzyme found in saliva and pancreatic fluid that breaks down fats into more simple forms for absorption by the gastrointestinal tract.

lipolysis. Breakdown of fats. In times of low blood sugar, lipolysis is the metabolic pathway that allows gluconeogenesis via ketosis. This is the inverse of fat storage that occurs in the presence of high blood glucose and insulin.

lokahi. Hawaiian word for unity, harmony, and balance.

loss of heterozygosity. A term describing the loss of the sole functioning, usually "wild type" allele that occurs via mutation, potentially resulting in the expression of a disease condition in that cell's lineage going forward. If an autosomal recessive trait is silent with one healthy "wild type" gene, then loss of heterozygosity can cause full disease expression.

lossy. A borrowed term from electrical engineering. In the context of information copying, if predictable loss of integrity occurs, the process is deemed to be "lossy."

leukocyte telomere length (LTL). The length of telomeres measured from white blood cells, or leukocytes. Often expressed in base pairs. The current technology provides averages, not specific information on critically short telomeres, and therefore is of limited use. In general, LTL decreases over a lifetime. The ease of LTL measurement has made this the unfortunate measurement of choice for researchers looking at general lifestyle and specific diseases with regard to telomere and telomerase function.

macular degeneration. A loss of central (macular) visual acuity that occurs and tends to progress with advanced age. Multifactorial with various degrees of genetic predisposition, this condition, along with Alzheimer's disease and hypertension, may be the result of an imbalance of retinal stem cell maintenance, destruction, and replacement.

mad cow disease. A transmissible, fatal neurological disease in cattle caused by an abnormally folding prion, or shape mimicry protein.

magnetic resonance imaging (MRI). An imaging technology that uses magnetic fields, other energy waves, and contrast media to create detailed images of internal organs. Because different tissues such as water and fat resonate differently to magnetic resonance, detailed images without ionizing radiation can be obtained.

maltose. A double sugar composed of two glucose molecules that is prevalent. This highly glycemic sugar is the breakdown product of germinating seeds, or malt, and is present in beer and artificially sweetened foods (see *glycemic index*).

Maslow's hierarchy of needs. A frequently taught psychological theory proposed by Abraham Maslow that suggests humans act according to a defined set of needs or objectives. These range from physiological and safety concerns to love and self-esteem and up to self-actualization and self-transcendence.

materialism. In philosophy, the belief that nothing exists except matter in its various states. Materialism often holds that concepts such as consciousness and spirit are unreal.

Mediterranean diet. A general description, based on the historical eating habits of peoples living around the Mediterranean Sea. Research suggests that these eating habits are associated with health advantages. This diet emphasizes limited red meat consumption, olive or canola oil over butter, spices over salt, and mainly consists of fruits, vegetables, whole grains, legumes, and nuts.

melatonin. A hormone produced by the pineal gland that regulates sleep and wakefulness cycles. It is also responsible for entraining the circadian rhythm and is therefore a *zeitgeber* (German for "time giver"). For jet lag, short-term melatonin use may be helpful in conjunction with light entrainment to the new time zone, although long-term use is not recommended.

Mendelian genetics. The science of gene inheritance discovered by Gregor Mendel that is the basis for our understanding of genetic heredity as it relates to discrete inheritable traits expressed by maternal and paternal variants of alleles, or genes.

mesenchymal stem cells (MSCs). A class of stem cells that maintain the capacity to differentiate into a wide variety of other stem cells. Mesenchymal stem cells are what enable the replenishment of regionally specific stem cells and they receive their more specialized programming largely from the surrounding milieu into which they are recruited.

messenger RNA (mRNA). A single-stranded discrete RNA polymer that carries a message that is first transcribed from a gene, leaves the nucleus, and then can be translated by ribosomes into a specific sequence of amino acids known as a protein (see *gene transcription* and *gene or mRNA translation*).

metabolic syndrome (syndrome X). A poorly defined yet prevalent condition of unbalanced health and metabolism. It is characterized by obesity, insulin resistance and high glucose, high blood pressure, high serum fats, and fatty liver. There are likely many pathways to metabolic syndrome, ranging from the molecular (see *adiponectin*), hormonal (see *ghrelin*), and functional, such as endocannabinoid deficiency, stress, inflammation, and aging itself.

mirror neurons. A functional class of brain cells, or neurons, that permits abstract identification with observed or imagined other (or self). When a monkey sees, the monkey's mirror neurons generate a mirrored version. The ability to generate a mirrored experience is important to empathy, self-insight, and the theory of mind.

monosaccharides. Organic molecules, usually with five or six carbons, that taste sweet and form the basis for cellular energy storage and utilization. A universal monosaccharide that is central to metabolism is glucose.

mosaic. When an organism contains different versions of the genetic code (see *genome*) in various cells, it is referred to as mosaic, just as a tile floor pattern can be composed of different shapes and colors of tile. Although chimeras (mixtures of species) and identical twins who shared stem cells across a placenta are obvious examples of mosaicism, in truth, DNA replication is lossy and all organisms are constantly generating low levels of mosaicism via chromothripsis and telomere erosion (see *lossy* and *chromothripsis*).

motherboard. In computers, this printed circuit board is home to the principal components of a computer, such as CPU, memory, input/output controllers, and other specialized "daughter" cards that can fit into slots on the motherboard.

mRNA or gene translation. The process by which mRNA is fed into ribosomes to be "read" and translated into a discrete chain of amino acids that will fold into a protein. The process uses tRNA (transfer RNA) to match the codon of the three nucleotide message (mRNA) to the anticodon of a specific tRNA amino acid carrier.

myelin. A fatty white layer that forms an electrically insulating sheath around the nerve transmitting extensions of neurons, called axons. The myelin is synthesized by supporting cells known as glial cells. Diets rich in essential fatty acids and vitamin B12 may assist in resisting demyelination conditions and frank diseases like multiple sclerosis.

NADH. A coenzyme with redox properties that is used by important cellular metabolic reactions such as glycolysis, the Krebs cycle, and the electron transport chain.

nasal turbinates. Intricate, bony, mucus-lined ridges on the inside of the nose that warm and moisturize air as well as trap airborne molecules.

niche. An abstract concept for the region around a stem cell surrounded by differentiated daughter cells that originated from that mother stem cell and therefore inherit many of her traits, including DNA errors and telomere lengths, as well as many epigenetic features that don't confer stemness (see *stemness* and *asymmetric division*).

non-REM Stage 1 (NREM1). A relatively short and light phase of sleep that serves as a transition down to deeper sleep (non-REM 2 or 3) or up to REM sleep or wakefulness. During NREM1, the sleeper's heart rate, breathing, and brain waves slow to alpha or theta waves and there can be hallucinations and twitching.

non-REM Stage 2 (NREM2). A transitional stage of sleep down to deeper NREM3 or up to lighter NREM1 that constitutes up to 50 percent of total sleep time. During this phase, theta wave activity around 6 to 10 cycles per second dominates with bursts of sleep spindles and K-complexes that may play a part in new neural pathway formations and declarative memory (see *sleep spindles* and *declarative memory*).

non-REM Stage 3 (NREM3). NREM3 is the deepest stage of sleep and occurs more in the first few cycles of sleep as opposed to the later cycles of an evening's rest. It is characterized by lack of dreaming and conscious awareness, and by slow delta waves (hence it is also called SWS, or slow wave sleep). During NREM3, many of the physical repairs occur as growth hormone peaks and cell replication is prioritized.

nucleus. A single spherical organelle present in most eukaryotic cells, protected by a double membrane with pores for access. The nucleus contains the genetic material known as chromosomes (see *chromosomes*).

obstructive sleep apnea. A very common collapse of the soft tissues of the upper respiratory system that produces obstruction, snoring, and inability to breathe while sleeping. The resulting hypopneas (or lack of breathing) cause frequent awakenings and interfere with restful and restorative sleep.

Occam's razor. A principle named after the English Scholasticism philosopher William of Occam that suggests that the fewer and simpler explanations you invoke to explain something, the more reliable your logic should be.

Okazaki fragments. Relatively short complementary DNA segments that assemble on the lagging strand. Due to the 5'→3' direction of DNA assembly, 5'→3' Okazaki fragments must be started with an RNA primer; those primers are later replaced with DNA in the splicing of adjacent fragments needed to form a continuous, complementary antisense or leading strand.

omega-3 fatty acids. A class of fats that have a double bond at the third carbon position. These important fatty acids cannot be synthesized and must be ingested from plant and marine sources. Omega-3 fatty acids are critical for a wide range of metabolic and synthetic functions.

oncogene. A gene that is typically involved in genetic surveillance, repair, or maintenance, cell cycle regulation and apoptosis, or contact inhibition (the inability to infringe on neighboring cells). When populations are inbred, abnormal variants of these oncogenes can result in suboptimal gene dosages of these cancer-preventing genes. In the course of mutation, as can occur from telomere erosion, loss of heterozygosity in any stem cell can result in a stem cell line prone to manifest as cancer.

opioids. Substances, both internally generated and externally ingested (from plants or pharmacological sources), that interact with opioid receptors to cause euphoria, pain relief, and other side effects.

organelles. Intracellular compartments or structures, often bound by their own membranes, that serve a purpose. Examples include the nucleus, which houses the genome; the mitochondria, which produce energy; lysosomes, which break down waste products; and the Golgi apparatus, responsible for packaging proteins and lipids into vesicles.

oxidation. The loss of electrons from one molecule (the oxidized) to another (the electron-accepting oxidizing agent). Always paired with reduction (see *REDOX*).

oxidative phosphorylation. A process that uses the electron transport chain in the mitochondria to make ATP. Transfer of electrons from NADH or FADH2 to O_2 creates a higher proton gradient outside the inner mitochondrial membrane; the flow of those protons back into the matrix is what powers ATP synthase to convert ADP into ATP (see *ATP* and *ATP synthase*).

p value. The probability value of a statistical result being merely the result of random chance. For example, a p value of 0.01 indicates a one percent chance of spurious association whereas a p value of 0.00001 indicates a one in 100,000 chance, or a very low probability that the association is not observable and therefore valid under the same conditions.

p53. Aka tumor suppressor p53, this is an enzyme known for its role as "the watchman of the genome." Its roles include initiating DNA repair, halting cell cycle progression (and therefore replication) if the chromosomes are aneuploid, and triggering cell suicide (apoptosis) if it deems the chromosomes beyond repair (see *apoptosis* and *double strand breakage repair*).

pancreas. A glandular organ behind the stomach that serves to control blood glucose and aid in digestion. It releases insulin to store glucose as fat when glucose is abundant and releases glucagon to signal fat breakdown when blood glucose is low. It also produces acid-neutralizing bicarbonate and food-digesting amylase, lipase, and protease into the duodenum via the ampulla of Vater (see *gluconeogenesis*).

parasomnias. Disorders of sleep generally associated with deep, slow-wave NREM3 sleep (although REM sleep parasomnias such as acting out dream content can occur). Parasomnias take forms including sleep talking, sleepwalking, bed wetting, and night terrors; all share a dysregulation of arousal, motor function, or autonomic function during a time when the mind and body should be at complete rest.

parasympathetic nervous system. The relaxing or restorative part of the autonomic nervous system that causes the "rest and relax" response. it works both in cooperation with and in opposition to the sympathetic nervous system.

pH. A logarithmic numeric scale used to express the relative acidity or alkalinity of a fluid. The range is generally measured from 0 (most acidic) to 14 (most basic or alkaline) depending on the relative presence of protons (H+) or hydrogen atoms lacking an electron. Various chemical reactions require specific pH conditions for efficient operation.

photoaging. Aging of the skin produced by light, usually of the ionizing ultraviolet spectrum.

pituitary gland. A small area of the brain below and working with the hypothalamus to secrete important hormones controlling growth, blood pressure, sex organs, lactation, skin pigmentation, thyroid glands, water/salt concentration, temperature, and the bonding hormone oxytocin.

plasmids. Small, circular double-stranded DNA that exists outside of the chromosomal DNA. This circular DNA is normal in bacteria but can also exist in eukaryotic cells.

point mutation. A change in one or very few nucleotides that encode a gene, resulting in an mRNA transcript that will result in an altered or nonfunctioning protein when translated, assuming the point mutation doesn't result in complete nonviability of the mRNA transcript.

post-mitotic. A differentiated and mature cell that can no longer undergo cell division or mitosis. An example would be a neuron that is highly specialized for nerve conduction and is no longer capable of dividing into two. Contrast this with self-renewing stem cells (see *stem cells*).

presbyopia. Advanced age causes loss of lens elasticity that results in the lens's inability to become round and focus at close distances. This loss of close vision is correctable by refractive lenses such as reading glasses or bifocals that have a positive refractive index.

prions. Proteins that are capable of producing shape mimicry in other proteins. Abnormal variants can be transmitted and cause mad cow disease or a human equivalent condition. Normal prions are essential to memory formation and their dysfunction in fatal familial insomnia shows their importance for normal sleep and memory formation (see *fatal familial insomnia*).

probiotics. Microorganisms (usually bacteria) that are believed to have benefits when ingested or introduced into a host organism's ecology. While it is true that many bacteria do set up permanent and stable symbiotic relationships that serve a protective or even beneficial function, the use of probiotics for improvement of small intestinal health is questionable.

procedural memory. Also known as implicit memory, procedural memory comprises the subconscious processes of skills such as playing a guitar, being a good friend, or lifting an arm. Constructed meaning and narratives about abstract ideas are forms of procedural memory and are largely constructed by an active user experience of dreaming during REM sleep (see *REM sleep*).

progeria. An inherited genetic disorder characterized by accelerated aging and death at an early age. Many forms of this accelerated aging are due to the absence of two working alleles of TERC or TERT (see *alleles*, *TERC*, *TERT*, and *dyskeratosis congenita*).

proprioception. The ability to sense body parts' position in space and the amount of force required to maintain them in that position.

protease. A digestive enzyme found in saliva and pancreatic fluid that breaks down protein chains into amino acids for absorption by the gastrointestinal tract.

proteins. Nitrogenous organic compounds composed of one or more long chains of amino acids that are assembled according to rules of mRNA or gene translation. Proteins are an essential part of all living organisms due to a variety of structural and functional roles.

pyloric sphincter. A muscular sphincter that separates the acidic stomach from the basic duodenum. Poor function of this sphincter can result in erosive damage to the duodenum, or a duodenal ulcer.

quantum theory. A branch of physics that attempts to explain more fundamental workings of reality at a relatively small and irreducible scale. In doing so, it embraces various ideas that seem absurd on a mundane level, such as nonduality, uncertainty of location, observations retroactively changing outcomes, and interactions between things at impossibly long distances.

rabbit starvation. Also known as protein poisoning, this form of malnutrition comes from a dietary dependence on overly lean meat without fat or stored glycogen. The high ammonium load from the amino acids of lean meat causes headache, diarrhea, fatigue, low heart rate and blood pressure, and food cravings.

R.A.J. A mnemonic acronym created by the author to explain a process of handling challenging experiences in real time. The steps are asking "Was it real?", identifying the Automatic Negative Thought, and constructing an antidote belief (or Judo Move) that reframes the experience with gratitude.

random access memory (RAM). Typically, a form of volatile storage of information on integrated circuit chips that, in contrast to other data storage methods such as disc drives, is lost when power is turned off. It allows for storage and use of information on a short-term basis.

reactive oxygen species (ROS). Oxygen-containing molecules that can cause damage to proteins, RNA, DNA, and fatty acids by oxidation (taking away electrons). ROS play normal roles in cellular metabolic pathways and autophagy, and their excess production by mitochondria is normally handled by intracellular catalase, superoxide dismutase, and glutathione. The blaming of ROS for disease arises from the association of toxins and radiation to their temporary accumulation but since aging also causes cell death, mitochondrial lysis, and inflammation, the contribution of ROS to fundamental causation remains unclear.

red blood cells. Biconcave blood cells without a nucleus that contain hemoglobin, a metalloprotein that carries both oxygen, needed for cellular respiration and carbon dioxide, a by-product of cellular respiration. Blood is literally more red when saturated with oxygen from breathing and less red when returning from the body in the veins.

Redenbacher effect. A concept invented by the author to explain the relatively synchronous and unfortunate decline in cellular function and health that occurs in advanced age. Just as nothing appears to happen while microwave popcorn is heating until all the kernels start popping at once, the Redenbacher effect could be related to ongoing damage in various stem cell types and/or an aging of the common source of progenitors, such as the MSCs.

REDOX. An exchange of electrons between molecules in which electrons are lost (oxidation) to a reducing agent and electrons are gained (reduction) by an oxidizing agent. Changes in the number of electrons allow for the transfer of energy in biochemical reactions such as oxidative phosphorylation.

reduction. The gain of electrons by one molecule (the reduced) from another (the electron-donating reducing agent). Always paired with oxidation (see *REDOX*).

REM sleep. A sleep phase in mammals and birds characterized by low muscle activity, rapid eye movements, vivid dreaming, and procedural memory formation. During REM sleep, a virtual reality is created by the dreamer's mind, and emotionality and subjective experiences are generated and observed as breathing and heart rate changes associated with alpha brain wave activity (7.5 to 12.5 cycles per second).

replicative senescence. "Aging" of cells that occurs as an emergent property of the "end replication problem" and lack of telomerase activity in non-stem cells (see *Hayflick limit* and *telomerase*).

resveratrol. A plant compound produced in response to attacks from pathogens such as bacteria and fungi. It is present in low levels in red wine, and was at one time thought to be linked to longevity through sirtuin pathway activation—a connection that has largely been debunked.

reverse transcription. Because the Central Dogma of Molecular Biology says DNA is the basis for RNA transcription, the making of DNA telomere segments from an RNA template on the TERC molecule is called "reverse" transcription (see *mRNA transcription* and *TERC*)

ribonucleic acid (RNA). A water-soluble, single-stranded polymer of nucleotides. There are many forms of RNA, serving roles in carrying messages (mRNA), transferring amino acids (tRNA), and modifying gene expression (small interfering, or siRNA, and micro, or miRNA).

semicircular canals. A structure in the inner ear that detects motion and acceleration in three dimensions, such as nodding, tilting one's head to touch the shoulder, and rotating the head to look right or left. It serves to orient the person in space and detect movement and is thus important in proprioception and introception (see *proprioception* and *introception*).

senolytic. The ability to aid or accelerate destruction of older and presumably damaged cells. Certain molecules, largely by virtue of their actions on the mechanisms of apoptosis, can accelerate clearance of older, damaged cells (see *apoptosis*).

sense strand. The 5'→3', lagging, positive, or sense strand is the half of DNA that reads analogously to the mRNA transcript (5'→3'). Its matching sister strand must be assembled in segments, called Okazaki fragments, with the use of RNA primers; hence the process is said to "lag" when copying this half of the double helix.

Shiva. The god of destruction in Hinduism that forms one part of the three forms (or trimurti) along with Brahma the creator and Vishnu the preserver. Shiva is charged with destruction of evil, which protects the universe.

Siamese twins. Conjoined twins. Two separate organisms joined anatomically because of incomplete cell separation. Called "Siamese" because of two famous twins from Thailand (then Siam) who traveled with the P. T. Barnum circus in the 19th century.

signs. In the context of disease presentation, a sign is an observable feature or elicitable response that may indicate the presence of disease (contrast with *symptoms*).

sirtuins. A broad and diverse class of proteins that facilitate chemical reactions such as transfer of chemical groups. The sirtuin-longevity connection has been largely debunked by actual experiments (see *resveratrol*).

sleep spindles. A burst of 12- to 14-cycle-per-second activity lasting at least 0.5 seconds that appears during NREM2 sleep and is associated with new declarative memory formation. People with fatal familial insomnia cannot form these spindles and therefore do not reap the benefits of this and deeper NREM3 sleep (see *fatal familial insomnia*).

slow-twitch muscles. A type of muscle fiber specialized for longer-duration action, such as long-distance running, which requires sustained use and continuous aerobic activity (or oxygen consumption).

stem cells. Specialized cells that are capable of self-renewal and asymmetric division. Self-renewal occurs because of active telomere lengthening by reverse transcription by telomerase. Asymmetric division means making a perfect copy of a stem mother and a more differentiated daughter (see *reverse transcription* and *asymmetric division*).

stemness. An abstract concept for distinguishing stem cells and more differentiated cell types. Stemness is often characterized by two traits: self-renewal and asymmetric division.

sympathetic nervous system. The activating or excitatory part of the autonomic nervous system that causes the "fight-or-flight" response. It works both in cooperation and in opposition to the parasympathetic nervous system.

symptoms. A subjective condition or state experienced and reportable by a person that represents an unusual state or disease condition (contrast with *signs*).

TA-65. A proprietary molecule derived from astragalus by the Geron Corporation and proven to be a telomerase activator.

Task Manager. Function on a Windows computer that displays some of the current active processes, programs, and performance that are occurring and potentially slowing your computer's CPU and memory (see *Ctrl-Alt-Delete*).

telomerase. Also known as TERT or terminal transferase. This protein is produced mainly in stem cells and, when cooperating with TERC (or telomerase RNA component), actively adds specific telomere segments to the ends of telomeres in a process known as reverse transcription (see *reverse transcription*).

telomerase activation. A general term for the ability of cells, usually stem cells, to produce TERT and TERC and utilize them for active lengthening of telomeres that normally erode with each cell division due to replicative senescence (see *replicative senescence, TERT,* and *TERC*).

telomerase RNA component (TERC). Provides the RNA template for the appropriate DNA of telomeres to be assembled. Although there can be different numbers and sequences of the RNA and matching DNA of repeated segments of telomeres, all eukaryotic cells require TERC and TERT to cooperate in lengthening telomeres.

telomerase reverse transcriptase (TERT). Works with TERC to actively lengthen the telomeric DNA ends of linear chromosomes. This process of using an RNA template to lengthen DNA is referred to as reverse transcription. Telomerase in stem cells confers self-renewal and thereby delays harmful mutations caused by critically short telomeres.

telomeres. Repetitive DNA sequences on the ends of linear, eukaryotic chromosomes. They prevent the chromosomes from being inappropriately joined together (see *double strand breakage repair*).

tetrahydrocannabinol (THC). The principal psychoactive molecule in cannabis, or marijuana. THC binds to both CB1 and CB2 endocannabinoid receptors and produces a variety of effects, including euphoria. It shows promise in treating several refractory conditions, perhaps by its general endocannabinoid triggering (see *endocannabinoid*).

theory of mind. The ability to create a working model of mental states in oneself and others that considers different points of view. A child must develop this theory of mind to understand that beliefs, intentions, actions, and knowledge are subjective and cannot be fully and accurately inferred.

theta brain waves. Theta wave activity around 3 to 8 cycles per second occurs during NREM1 and NREM2 sleep and is characterized by a relaxed and suggestible frame of mind as well as intuition, emotionality, and creativity.

Tourette's. Aka Tourette's syndrome. A neuropsychiatric disorder of unknown origin that is characterized by tics, which are involuntary repetitive, nonrhythmic motor movements or vocalizations. In common usage, someone who uses profanity in an uncontrolled fashion is said to have Tourette's although this is a misconception.

transhumanism. An intellectual movement that broadly embraces technological modifications of human physiology and form for the stated purpose of longevity, intellectual capacity, and increased capabilities.

trimurti. The trimurti (three forms) of one version of Hindu theology usually includes Brahma, Vishnu, and Shiva (see *Brahma, Vishnu,* and *Shiva*).

Vishnu. The god of preservation in Hinduism that forms one part of the three forms (or trimurti) along with Brahma the creator and Shiva the destroyer. Vishnu in his incarnations, such as Lords Rama and Krishna, is tasked with bringing balance between good and evil during troubled times.

vitamin B12. A vitamin whose dietary deficiency causes low blood counts (anemia) and neurological problems. Unfortified pure plant diets are deficient in vitamin B12 and represent a preventable danger of this food regimen.

VO$_2$ max. The measurable sustainable peak oxygen utilization as measured during strenuous aerobic activity (such as running on a treadmill). The VO$_2$ max tends to measurably decrease as we age due to reduced cardiopulmonary capacity, reduced oxygen carrying by blood cells, and decreased oxygen requirements of slow-twitch muscles.

wild type. The most common and normally functioning variant of a gene in a species. Although certain genes such as those related to eye color confer no clear advantage, most alleles have a common and normally functioning "wild type" allele owing to common ancestry and competitive advantage in a genetically well-established species.

zygote. The diploid (46 chromosomes in humans) fertilized egg made from the fusion of a haploid egg and haploid sperm (haploid being half or 23 chromosomes).

ENDNOTES

Chapter 1: The Quest to End Aging

1. "The Nobel Prize in Physiology or Medicine 2009." *Nobelprize.org.* Nobel Media AB 2014. Web. 30 Aug 2017. http://www.nobelprize.org/nobel_prizes/medicine/laureates/2009/.

2. C. Schaefer, S. Sciortino, M. Kvale, et al. "B4-3: Demographic and Behavioral Influences on Telomere Length and Relationship with All-Cause Mortality: Early Results from the Kaiser Permanente Research Program on Genes, Environment, and Health (RPGEH)." *Clinical Medicine & Research* 11, no. 3 (September 2013): 146. doi:10.3121/cmr.2013.1176.b4-3.

3. R. M. Cawthon, K. R. Smith, E. O'Brien, et al. "Association between telomere length in blood and mortality in people aged 60 years or older." *The Lancet* 361, no. 9355 (February 1, 2003): 393-95. doi: http://dx.doi.org/10.1016/S0140-6736(03)12384-7.

4. A. L. Fitzpatrick, R. A. Kronmal, M. Kimura, et al. "Leukocyte Telomere Length and Mortality in the Cardiovascular Health Study." *The Journals of Gerontology Series A: Biological Sciences and Medical Sciences* 66A, no. 4 (April 2011): 421-29. doi:10.1093/gerona/glq224.

5. Line Rode, Børge G. Nordestgaard, and Stig E. Bojesen. "Peripheral Blood Leukocyte Telomere Length and Mortality Among 64 637 Individuals From the General Population." *JNCI: Journal of the National Cancer Institute* 107, no. 6 (June 1, 2015). doi:https://doi.org/10.1093/jnci/djv074.

6. M. Crous-Bou, T. T. Fung, J. Prescott, et al. "Mediterranean diet and telomere length in Nurses Health Study: population based cohort study." *British Medical Journal* 349 (December 02, 2014). doi:https://doi.org/10.1136/bmj.g6674.

7.   P. Sjögren, R. Fisher, L. Kallings, et al. "Stand up for health—avoiding sedentary behaviour might lengthen your telomeres: secondary outcomes from a physical activity RCT in older people." *British Journal of Sports Medicine* 48, no. 19 (October 03, 2014): 1407-409. doi:10.1136/bjsports-2013-093342.

8.   Aric A. Prather, Eli Puterman, Jue Lin, et al. "Shorter Leukocyte Telomere Length in Midlife Women with Poor Sleep Quality." *Journal of Aging Research* 2011 (October 20, 2011): 1-6. doi:10.4061/2011/721390.

9.   "QuickStats: Percentage Distribution of Deaths,* by Place of Death†,§— United States, 2000–2014." *MMWR. Morbidity and Mortality Weekly Report* 65, no. 13 (April 08, 2016): 357. doi:10.15585/mmwr.6513a6.

Chapter 2: Biology 101—Genetics and Cell Biology

1.   M. P. Baar, R. M. Brandt, and D. A. Putavet, "Targeted Apoptosis of Senescent Cells Restores Tissue Homeostasis in Response to Chemotoxicity and Aging," Cell 169, no. 1 (March 23, 2017): 132-147.

2.   "Genetics Home Reference: Your Guide to Understanding Genetic Conditions: What is DNA?" U.S. National Library of Medicine, August 29, 2017, accessed August 31, 2017, https://ghr.nlm.nih.gov/primer/basics/dna.

3.   H. J. Muller, 1938. The remaking of chromosomes. Collecting Net (Woods Hole) 13: 181–198.

4.   B. E. Flanary and G. Kletetschka, "Analysis of telomere length and telomerase activity in tree species of various life-spans, and with age in the bristlecone pine Pinus longaeva," *Biogerontology* 6, no. 2 (2005): 101-111, doi:10.1007/s10522-005-3484-4.

Chapter 3: Aging—One Cause, One Cure

1.   R. D. Semba, L. Ferrucci, and B. Bartali, "Resveratrol Levels and All-Cause Mortality in Older Community-Dwelling Adults," *JAMA Internal Medicine* 174, no. 7 (July 01, 2014): 1077-1084, doi:10.1001/jamainternmed.2014.1582.

2.   J. M. Van Raamsdonk and S. Hekimi, "Deletion of the Mitochondrial Superoxide Dismutase sod-2 Extends Lifespan in Caenorhabditis elegans," *PLoS Genetics* 5, no. 2 (February 06, 2009), doi:10.1371/journal.pgen.1000361.

3.   J. Viña, C. Borras, and K. M. Abdelaziz, "The Free Radical Theory of Aging Revisited: The Cell Signaling Disruption Theory of Aging," *Antioxidants & Redox Signaling* 19, no. 8 (September 10, 2013): 779-787, doi:10.1089/ars.2012.5111.

4.   E. Epel, J. Lin, F.H. Wilhelm, et al., "Cell aging in relation to stress arousal and cardiovascular disease risk factors," *Psychoneuroendocrinology* 31, no. 3 (November 17, 2006): 277-287, doi:10.1016/j.psyneuen.2005.08.011.

5. A. M. Valdes et al., "Obesity, cigarette smoking, and telomere length in women," *The Lancet* 366, no. 9486 (June 14, 2005): 662-664, doi:10.1016/s0140-6736(05)66630-5.

6. M. Harbo, L. Bendix, A. C. Bay-Jensen et al., "The distribution pattern of critically short telomeres in human osteoarthritic knees," *Arthritis Research & Therapy* 14, no. 1 (January 18, 2012), doi:10.1186/ar3687.

7. A. M. Valdes, J. B. Richards, J. P. Gardner et al., "Telomere length in leukocytes correlates with bone mineral density and is shorter in women with osteoporosis," *Osteoporosis International* 18, no. 9 (March 09, 2007): 1203-1210, doi:10.1007/s00198-007-0357-5.

8. M. Jaskelioff, F. L. Muller, J. H. Paik et al., "Telomerase reactivation reverses tissue degeneration in aged telomerase-deficient mice," *Nature* 469, no. 7328 (November 28, 2010): 102-106, doi:10.1038/nature09603.

9. G. Atzmon, M. Cho, R. M. Cawthon et al., "Genetic variation in human telomerase is associated with telomere length in Ashkenazi centenarians," *Proceedings of the National Academy of Sciences* 107, no. Suppl_1 (November 13, 2009), doi:10.1073/pnas.0906191106.

Chapter 4: Your Breath

1. M. Y. Armanios, J. J. L. Chen, J. D. Cogan et al., "Telomerase Mutations in Families with Idiopathic Pulmonary Fibrosis," *New England Journal of Medicine* 356, no. 13 (March 29, 2007): 1317-1326, doi:10.1056/nejmoa066157.

2. S. E. Stanley, J. J. Chen, J. D. Podlevsky et al., "Telomerase mutations in smokers with severe emphysema," *Journal of Clinical Investigation* 125, no. 2 (December 22, 2014): 563-570, doi:10.1172/jci78554.

3. L. Rode, S. E. Bojesen, M. Weischer et al., "Short telomere length, lung function and chronic obstructive pulmonary disease in 46,396 individuals," *Thorax* 68, no. 5 (December 25, 2012): 429-435, doi:10.1136/thoraxjnl-2012-202544.

4. E. Albrecht, E. Sillanpää, S. Karrasch et al., "Telomere length in circulating leukocytes is associated with lung function and disease," *European Respiratory Journal* 43, no. 4 (December 5, 2013): 983-992, doi:10.1183/09031936.00046213.

5. C. J. Saux, P. Davy, and C. Brampton, "A Novel Telomerase Activator Suppresses Lung Damage in a Murine Model of Idiopathic Pulmonary Fibrosis," *PLoS ONE* 8, no. 3 (March 14, 2013), doi:10.1371/journal.pone.0058423.

Chapter 5: Your Mind

1. M. Brüne and U. Brüne-Cohrs, "Theory of mind—evolution, ontogeny, brain mechanisms and psychopathology," *Neuroscience & Biobehavioral Reviews* 30, no. 4 (October 18, 2006): 437-455, doi:10.1016/j.neubiorev.2005.08.001.

2. M. Iacoboni, R. P. Woods, M. Brass et al., "Cortical Mechanisms of Human Imitation," *Science* 286, no. 5449 (December 24, 1999): 2526-2528, doi:10.1126/science.286.5449.2526.

3. L. Fadiga, L. Fogassi, G. Pavesi et al., "Motor facilitation during action observation: a magnetic stimulation study," *Journal of Neurophysiology* 27, no. 6 (June 1, 1995): 2608-2611.

4. L. M. Oberman and V. S. Ramachandran, "Broken Mirrors: A Theory of Autism," *Scientific American* 295, no. 5 (June 1, 2007): 62-69, doi:10.1038/scientificamerican1106-62.

5. NCI Staff, "Antioxidants Accelerate the Growth and Invasiveness of Tumors in Mice," *National Cancer Institute* April 12, 2015, accessed August 31, 2017, https://www.cancer.gov/news-events/cancer-currents-blog/2015/antioxidants-metastasis.

6. H. G. Prigerson, Y. Bao, M. A. Shah et al., "Chemotherapy Use, Performance Status, and Quality of Life at the End of Life," *JAMA Oncology* 1, no. 6 (September 01, 2015): 778-784, doi:10.1001/jamaoncol.2015.2378.

7. Marcia Angell, *The Truth About the Drug Companies: How they deceive us and what to do about it* (Melbourne: Scribe, 2006).

8. J. Choi, S. R. Fauce, and R. B. Effros, "Reduced telomerase activity in human T lymphocytes exposed to cortisol," *Brain, Behavior, and Immunity* 22, no. 4 (January 25, 2008): 600-605, doi:10.1016/j.bbi.2007.12.004.

9. E. S. Epel, E. H. Blackburn, J. Lin et al., "Accelerated telomere shortening in response to life stress," *Proceedings of the National Academy of Sciences* 101, no. 49 (December 01, 2004): 17312-17315, doi:10.1073/pnas.0407162101.

10. D. Ornish, J. Lin, J. M. Chan et al., "Effect of comprehensive lifestyle changes on telomerase activity and telomere length in men with biopsy-proven low-risk prostate cancer: 5-year follow-up of a descriptive pilot study," *The Lancet Oncology* 14, no. 11 (September 17, 2013): 1112-1120, doi:10.1016/s1470-2045(13)70366-8.

11. D. H. Rehkopf, W. H. Dow, L. Rosero-Bixby et al., "Longer leukocyte telomere length in Costa Ricas Nicoya Peninsula: A population-based study," *Experimental Gerontology* 48, no. 11 (August 27, 2013): 1266-1273, doi:10.1016/j.exger.2013.08.005.

12. J. Daubenmier, J. Lin, E. Blackburn et al., "Changes in stress, eating, and metabolic factors are related to changes in telomerase activity in a randomized mindfulness intervention pilot study," *Psychoneuroendocrinology*

37, no. 7 (December 14, 2012): 917-928, doi:10.1016/j. psyneuen.2011.10.008.

13. M. Wikgren, M. Maripuu, T. Karlsson et al., "Short Telomeres in Depression and the General Population Are Associated with a Hypocortisolemic State," *Biological Psychiatry* 71, no. 4 (November 4, 2012): 294-300, doi:10.1016/j. biopsych.2011.09.015.

14. Mihaly Csikszentmihalyi, TED: Ideas worth spreading, February 2004, accessed August 31, 2017, https://www.ted.com/talks/ mihaly_csikszentmihalyi_on_flow.

Chapter 6: Your Sleep

1. L. Xie, H. Kang, Q. Xu et al., "Sleep Drives Metabolite Clearance from the Adult Brain," *Science* 342, no. 6156 (October 17, 2013): 373-377, doi:10.1126/ science.1241224.

2. Marta Jackowska, Mark Hamer, and Livia A. Carvalho, "Short Sleep Duration Is Associated with Shorter Telomere Length in Healthy Men: Findings from the Whitehall II Cohort Study," *PLoS ONE* 7, no. 10 (October 29, 2012), doi:10.1371/journal.pone.0047292.

3. K. A. Lee, C. Gay, J. Humphreys et al., "Telomere Length is Associated with Sleep Duration But Not Sleep Quality in Adults with Human Immunodeficiency Virus," *Sleep* 37, no. 1 (January 2014): 157-166, doi:10.5665/sleep.3328.

4. A. Rechtschaffen and B. M. Bergmann, "Sleep Deprivation in the Rat: An Update of the 1989 Paper," *Sleep* 25, no. 1 (February 2002): 18-24, doi:10.1093/sleep/25.1.18.

5. Y. Yeo, S. H. Ma, S. K. Park et al., "A Prospective Cohort Study on the Relationship of Sleep Duration With All-cause and Disease-specific Mortality in the Korean Multi-center Cancer Cohort Study," *Journal of Preventive Medicine & Public Health* 46, no. 5 (September 30, 2013): 271-281, doi:10.3961/jpmph.2013.46.5.271.

6. J. Orzeł-Gryglewska, "Consequences of sleep deprivation," *International Journal of Occupational Medicine and Environmental Health* 23, no. 1 (2010): 95-114, doi:10.2478/v10001-010-0004-9.

7. C. Fernandes, N. B. Rocha, S. Rocha et al., "Detrimental role of prolonged sleep deprivation on adult neurogenesis," *Frontiers in Cellular Neuroscience* 9, no. 140 (April 14, 2015), doi:10.3389/fncel.2015.00140.

8. D. Dunning, K. Johnson, J. Ehrlinger et al., "Why People Fail to Recognize Their Own Incompetence," *Current Directions in Psychological Science* 12, no. 3 (June 1, 2003): 83-87, doi:10.1111/1467-8721.01235.

9. "1 in 3 adults don't get enough sleep," CDC Newsroom, February 18, 2016, accessed September 01, 2017, https://www.cdc.gov/media/releases/2016/p0215-enough-sleep.html.

10. B. Rasch, C. Buchel, S. Gais et al., "Odor Cues During Slow-Wave Sleep Prompt Declarative Memory Consolidation," *Science* 315, no. 5817 (March 09, 2007): 1326-1429, doi:10.1126/science.1138581.

11. J. F. Garvey, M. F. Pengo, P. Drakoatos et al., "Epidemiological aspects of obstructive sleep apnea.," *Journal of Thoracic Disease* 7, no. 5 (May 2015): 920-929, doi:10.3978/j.issn.2072-1439.2015.04.52.

12. L. L. Von Moltke and D. J. Greenblatt, "Medication dependence and anxiety," *Dialogues in Clinical Neuroscience* 5, no. 3 (September 2003): 237-245.

13. "Melatonin," University of Maryland Medical Center, 2013, accessed September 01, 2017, http://www.umm.edu/Health/Medical/AltMed/Supplement/Melatonin.

14. J. K. M. Chan, J. Trinder, I. M. Colrain et al., "The Acute Effects of Alcohol on Sleep Electroencephalogram Power Spectra in Late Adolescence," *Alcoholism: Clinical and Experimental Research* 39, no. 2 (January 16, 2015): 291-299, doi:10.1111/acer.12621.

15. M. Jackowska, M. Hamer, L. A. Carvalho et al., "Short Sleep Duration Is Associated with Shorter Telomere Length in Healthy Men: Findings from the Whitehall II Cohort Study," *PLoS ONE* 7, no. 10 (October 29, 2012): e47292, doi:10.1371/journal.pone.0047292.

16. M. R. Cribbet, M. Carlisle, R. M. Cawthon et al., "Cellular Aging and Restorative Processes: Subjective Sleep Quality and Duration Moderate the Association between Age and Telomere Length in a Sample of Middle-Aged and Older Adults," *Sleep* 37, no. 1 (January 2014): 65-70, doi:10.5665/sleep.3308.

17. K. Savolainen, J. G. Eriksson, E. Kajantie et al., "The history of sleep apnea is associated with shorter leukocyte telomere length: the Helsinki Birth Cohort Study," *Sleep Medicine* 15, no. 2 (February 2014): 209-212, doi:10.1016/j.sleep.2013.11.779.

18. A. Barceló, J. Piérola, H. López-Escribano et al., "Telomere shortening in sleep apnea syndrome," *Respiratory Medicine* 104, no. 8 (August 2010): 1225-1229, doi:10.1016/j.rmed.2010.03.025.

Chapter 7: Your Exercise

1. D. Sagoe, H. Molde, C. S. Andreassen et al., "The global epidemiology of anabolic-androgenic steroid use: a meta-analysis and meta-regression analysis," *Annals of Epidemiology* 24, no. 5 (May 2014): 383-398, doi:10.1016/j.annepidem.2014.01.009.

2. C. Ballantyne, "Follow Your Own Rules To Crush Life," *Roman Fitness Systems* (web blog), 2014, accessed September 1, 2017, http://romanfitnesssystems. com/articles/your-rules/.

3. D. Dlouha, J. Maluskova, I. Kralova Lesna, et al., "Comparison of the relative telomere length measured in leukocytes and eleven different human tissues," *Physiological Research* 63, no. Suppl 3 (July 8, 2014): S343-S350.

4. M. Kveiborg, M. Kassem, B. Langdahl et al., "Telomere shortening during aging of human osteoblasts in vitro and leukocytes in vivo: lack of excessive telomere loss in osteoporotic patients," *Mechanisms of Ageing and Development* 106, no. 3 (January 15, 1999): 261-271, doi:10.1016/s0047-6374(98)00114-6.

5. J. Z. Guan, W. P. Guan, T. Maeda et al., "Different levels of hypoxia regulate telomere length and telomerase activity," *Aging Clinical and Experimental Research* 24, no. 3 (June 2012): 213-217, doi:10.1007/bf03325250.

6. D. G. Chang, J. A. Holt, and M. Sklar, "Yoga as a treatment for chronic low back pain: A systematic review of the literature," *Journal of Orthopedics & Rheumatology* 3, no. 1 (January 1, 2016): 1-8, doi:10.13188/2334-2846.1000018.

7. E. Mundstock, H. Zatti, and F. M. Louzada, "Effects of physical activity in telomere length: Systematic review and meta-analysis," *Ageing Research Reviews* 22 (July 2015): 72-80, doi:10.1016/j.arr.2015.02.004.

8. P. D. Loprinzi, J. P. Loenneke, and E. H. Blackburn, "Movement-Based Behaviors and Leukocyte Telomere Length among US Adults," *Medicine & Science in Sports & Exercise* 47, no. 11 (November 2015): 2747-2752, doi:10.1249/mss.0000000000000695.

9. D. Saßenroth, A. Meyer, B. Salewsky et al., "Sports and Exercise at Different Ages and Leukocyte Telomere Length in Later Life – Data from the Berlin Aging Study II (BASE-II)," *Plos One* 10, no. 12 (December 02, 2015): e0142131, doi:10.1371/journal.pone.0142131.

10. M. K. Laine, J. G. Eriksson, U. M. Kujala et al., "Effect of intensive exercise in early adult life on telomere length in later life in men. Laine MK," *Journal of Sports Science & Medicine* 14, no. 2 (May 8, 2015): 239-245.

11. L. Soares-Miranda, F. Imamura, D. Siscovick et al., "Physical Activity, Physical Fitness, and Leukocyte Telomere Length," *Medicine & Science in Sports & Exercise* 47, no. 12 (December 2015), doi:10.1249/mss.0000000000000720.

12. M. Collins, V. Renault, L. A. Grobler et al, "Athletes with Exercise-Associated Fatigue Have Abnormally Short Muscle DNA Telomeres," *Medicine & Science in Sports & Exercise* 35, no. 9 (September 2003): 1524-1528, doi:10.1249/01. mss.0000084522.14168.49.

Chapter 8: Your Diet

1. J. LaLanne, "Quotes," Jack Lalanne, Page 191, accessed September 01, 2017, http://jacklalanne.com/quotes/.

2. M. Crous-Bou, T. T. Fung, J. Prescott et al., "Mediterranean diet and telomere length in Nurses Health Study: population based cohort study," *BMJ* 349, no. G6674 (December 02, 2014), doi:10.1136/bmj.g6674.

3. S. Garcia-Calzon, G. Zalba, M. Ruiz-Canela et al., "Dietary inflammatory index and telomere length in subjects with a high cardiovascular disease risk from the PREDIMED-NAVARRA study: cross-sectional and longitudinal analyses over 5 y," *American Journal of Clinical Nutrition* 102, no. 4 (October 09, 2015): 897-904, doi:10.3945/ajcn.115.116863.

4. V. Boccardi, A. Esposito, M. R. Rizzo et al., "Mediterranean Diet, Telomere Maintenance and Health Status among Elderly," *PLoS ONE* 8, no. 4 (April 30, 2013): 1-6, doi:10.1371/journal.pone.0062781.

5. M. Zhou, L. Zhu, X. Cui et al., "Influence of diet on leukocyte telomere length, markers of inflammation and oxidative stress in individuals with varied glucose tolerance: a Chinese population study," *Nutrition Journal*15, no. 1 (April 12, 2015), doi:10.1186/s12937-016-0157-x.

6. S. Garcia-Calzon, G. Zalba, M. Ruiz-Canela et al., "Dietary inflammatory index and telomere length in subjects with a high cardiovascular disease risk from the PREDIMED-NAVARRA study: cross-sectional and longitudinal analyses over 5 y," *American Journal of Clinical Nutrition* 102, no. 4 (October 09, 2015): 897-904, doi:10.3945/ajcn.115.116863.

7. A. M. Valdes, T. Andrew, and J. P. Gardner, "Obesity, cigarette smoking, and telomere length in women," *The Lancet* 366, no. 9486 (August 2005): 662-664, doi:10.1016/s0140-6736(05)66630-5.

8. J. Daubenmier, J. Lin, and E. Blackburn, "Changes in stress, eating, and metabolic factors are related to changes in telomerase activity in a randomized mindfulness intervention pilot study," *Psychoneuroendocrinology* 37, no. 7 (July 2012): 917-928, doi:10.1016/j.psyneuen.2011.10.008.

Chapter 9: Your Supplements

1. "Top-selling vitamin supplements investigated Are they worth taking?" review, *Consumer Reports* (web log), June 2011, accessed September 1, 2017, https://www.consumerreports.org/cro/2012/04/top-selling-vitamin-supplements/index.htm.

2. "Vitamins," MedlinePlus Medical Encyclopedia, August 16, 2017, accessed September 01, 2017, https://medlineplus.gov/ency/article/002399.htm.

3. D. Harvie, *Limeys: The True Story of One Man's War against Ignorance, the Establishment and the Deadly Scurvy* (The History Press, 2005).

4. A. Hawk, "The Great Disease Enemy, Kakke (Beriberi) and the Imperial Japanese Army," *Military Medicine* 171, no. 4 (April 2006): 333-339, doi:10.7205/milmed.171.4.333.

5. J. Mursu, K. Robien, L. J. Harnack et al, "Dietary Supplements and Mortality Rate in Older Women," *Archives of Internal Medicine* 171, no. 18 (October 10, 2011): 1625-1633, doi:10.1001/archinternmed.2011.445.

6. Y. Zhang, Y. Ikeno, W. Qi et al., "Mice Deficient in Both Mn Superoxide Dismutase and Glutathione Peroxidase-1 Have Increased Oxidative Damage and a Greater Incidence of Pathology but No Reduction in Longevity," *The Journals of Gerontology Series A: Biological Sciences and Medical Sciences* 64A, no. 12 (December 23, 2009): 1212-1220, doi:10.1093/gerona/glp132.

7. "Coenzyme Q10," University of Maryland Medical Center, accessed September 1, 2017, http://umm.edu/health/medical/altmed/supplement/coenzyme-q10.

8. "Coenzyme Q10 Evidence," Mayo Clinic, November 01, 2013, accessed September 01, 2017, http://www.mayoclinic.org/drugs-supplements/coenzyme-q10/evidence/hrb-20059019.

9. M. E. Madmani, A. Y. Solaiman, and K. T. Agha, "Coenzyme Q10 for heart failure," *Cochrane Database of Systematic Reviews* 6 (June 02, 2014), doi:10.1002/14651858.cd008684.pub2.

10. M. J. Ho, E. C. Li, and J. M. Wright, "Blood pressure lowering efficacy of coenzyme Q10 for primary hypertension," *Cochrane Database of Systematic Reviews* 3, no. CD007435 (March 03, 2016), doi:10.1002/14651858.cd007435.pub3.

11. P. J. Skerrett, "Resveratrol-the hype continues," Harvard Health Blog, February 03, 2012, accessed September 01, 2017, https://www.health.harvard.edu/blog/resveratrol-the-hype-continues-201202034189.

12. H. H. Floch, W. A. Walker, S. Guandalini et al., "Recommendations for Probiotic Use—2008 Response," *Journal of Clinical Gastroenterology* 43, no. 8 (July 2009): S104-S108, doi:10.1097/mcg.0b013e31819e8be3.

13. J. Walter, "Ecological Role of Lactobacilli in the Gastrointestinal Tract: Implications for Fundamental and Biomedical Research," *Applied and Environmental Microbiology* 74, no. 16 (August 06, 2008): 4985-4996, doi:10.1128/aem.00753-08.

14. "Coenzyme Q10 Evidence," Mayo Clinic, November 01, 2013, accessed September 01, 2017, http://www.mayoclinic.org/drugs-supplements/coenzyme-q10/evidence/hrb-20059019.

15. Harvard Health Publications, "Growth hormone, athletic performance, and aging," Harvard Health, May 2010, accessed September 01,

2017, https://www.health.harvard.edu/diseases-and-conditions/growth-hormone-athletic-performance-and-aging.

16. D.C. Lee, J.A. Im, J.H. Kim et al., "Effect of Long-Term Hormone Therapy on Telomere Length in Postmenopausal Women," *Yonsei Medical Journal* 46, no. 4 (August 2005): 471-479, doi:10.3349/ymj.2005.46.4.471.

17. D. M. Townsley, B. Dumitriu, and D. Liu, "Danazol Treatment for Telomere Diseases," *New England Journal of Medicine* 374, no. 20 (May 19, 2016): 1922-1931, doi:10.1056/nejmoa1515319.

18. B. Molgora, R. Bateman, G. Sweeney et al., "Functional Assessment of Pharmacological Telomerase Activators in Human T Cells," *Cells* 2, no. 1 (January 14, 2013): 57-66, doi:10.3390/cells2010057.

19. P. Willeit, J. Willeit, A. Mayr et al., "Telomere Length and Risk of Incident Cancer and Cancer Mortality," *Jama* 304, no. 1 (July 07, 2010): 69-75, doi:10.1001/jama.2010.897.

20. J. Mursu, K. Robien, L. J. Harnack et al., "Dietary Supplements and Mortality Rate in Older Women," *Archives of Internal Medicine* 171, no. 18 (October 10, 2011): 1625-1633, doi:10.1001/archinternmed.2011.445.

21. C. Wary, C. Brillault-Salvat, and G. Bloch, "Effect of chronic magnesium supplementation on magnesium distribution in healthy volunteers evaluated by 31P-NMRS and ion selective electrodes," *British Journal of Clinical Pharmacology* 48, no. 5 (November 24, 2001): 655-662, doi:10.1046/j.1365-2125.1999.00063.x

Chapter 10: What Do You See in Your TeloMirrors?

1. "Abraham Maslow," Pursuit of Happiness, September 10, 2016, accessed September 01, 2017, http://www.pursuit-of-happiness.org/history-of-happiness/abraham-maslow/.

2. A. H. Maslow, *The Farther Reaches of Human Nature* (New York: Penguin Group, 1993).

3. M. E. Koltko-Rivera, "Rediscovering the later version of Maslow's hierarchy of needs: Self-transcendence and opportunities for theory, research, and unification," *Review of General Psychology* 10, no. 4 (December 2006): 302-317, doi:10.1037/1089-2680.10.4.302

Chapter 12: The Future Is Ageless

1. J. Krakauer, "Lost in the Wild: On April 28, 24-year-old Chris McCandless walked off into America's Last Frontier, hoping to make sense of his life. Four months later, he was dead. This is his story." *Outside*, January 1993.

2. F. R. Shapiro, *Yale Book of Quotations* (Yale University Press, 2006), Hamlet, William Shakespeare, act 1, scene 1, 1.83 (1601).

INDEX

E

ACKNOWLEDGMENTS

I wish to acknowledge my family, friends, patients, subscribers to my blogs and YouTube channel, and even those who have been critical of my ideas.

I appreciate April Underwood for introducing me to Lindi Stolar, my book strategist. I'm also grateful for my literary agent, Steve Troha. Finally, this book would never have been possible without three key partners: my writer, Marianne Kotcher, my illustrator, Cecelia Snaith (www.ceceliasnaith.com), and my editor, Anne Barthel. Thank you all!

ABOUT THE AUTHOR

Ed Park, M.D., M.P.H., is a telomere and telomerase expert and founder of Recharge Biomedical. He received his undergraduate degree with honors from Harvard University in Anthropology; his M.D. is from Columbia University College of Physicians and Surgeons; and he earned a Masters of Public Health from Columbia University. He completed his internship and residency at Beth Israel Hospital, a teaching hospital of the Harvard Medical School, in 1997. Dr. Park was an attending physician in Obstetrics and Gynecology with Kaiser Permanente in Orange County, California, before practicing solo ob-gyn until 2010. In 2007 he became one of the first 20 people in the world to regularly ingest a nutraceutical telomerase activator, and he has taken no other supplements or medicines for over 10 years. In 2008 he became the first licensed M.D. to prescribe it, and began to report on his patients' amazing results via blogs and videos. Through this journey, Dr. Park has become a popular speaker, guest, and expert on aging generally and the sole evangelist in what he calls "Telomerase Activation Medicine."

Website: rechargebiomedical.com

Hay House Titles of Related Interest

YOU CAN HEAL YOUR LIFE, the movie, starring Louise Hay & Friends
(available as a 1-DVD program, an expanded 2-DVD set,
and an online streaming video)
Learn more at www.hayhouse.com/louise-movie

THE SHIFT, the movie,
starring Dr. Wayne W. Dyer
(available as a 1-DVD program, an expanded 2-DVD set,
and an online streaming video)
Learn more at www.hayhouse.com/the-shift-movie

———

*THE BIOLOGY OF BELIEF 10th ANNIVERSARY EDITION:
Unleashing the Power of Consciousness, Matter & Miracles,*
by Bruce H. Lipton, Ph.D.

*HUMAN BY DESIGN: From Evolution by Chance
to Transformation by Choice,*
by Gregg Braden

*THE MINDBODY SELF: How Longevity Is Culturally Learned
and the Causes of Health Are Inherited,*
by Dr. Mario Martinez

———

All of the above are available at your local bookstore,
or may be ordered by contacting Hay House (see next page)

We hope you enjoyed this Hay House book. If you'd like to receive our online catalog featuring additional information on Hay House books and products, or if you'd like to find out more about the Hay Foundation, please contact:

Hay House, Inc., P.O. Box 5100, Carlsbad, CA 92018-5100
(760) 431-7695 or (800) 654-5126
(760) 431-6948 (fax) or (800) 650-5115 (fax)
www.hayhouse.com® • www.hayfoundation.org

———

Published and distributed in Australia by:
Hay House Australia Pty. Ltd., 18/36 Ralph St., Alexandria NSW 2015
Phone: 612-9669-4299 • *Fax:* 612-9669-4144 • www.hayhouse.com.au

Published and distributed in the United Kingdom by:
Hay House UK, Ltd., Astley House, 33 Notting Hill Gate, London W11 3JQ
Phone: 44-20-3675-2450 • *Fax:* 44-20-3675-2451 • www.hayhouse.co.uk

Published in India by: Hay House Publishers India,
Muskaan Complex, Plot No. 3, B-2, Vasant Kunj, New Delhi 110 070
Phone: 91-11-4176-1620 • *Fax:* 91-11-4176-1630 • www.hayhouse.co.in

Distributed in Canada by:
Raincoast Books, 2440 Viking Way, Richmond, B.C. V6V 1N2
Phone: 1-800-663-5714 • *Fax:* 1-800-565-3770 • www.raincoast.com

———

Access New Knowledge.
Anytime. Anywhere.

Learn and evolve at your own pace
with the world's leading experts.

www.hayhouseU.com